The Genocide Principle

This book explores how and why genocide is a transcultural and transhistorical phenomenon, reflects the unconscious processes that drive human nature, and draws broadly on psychoanalytic theory, as well as on social science and philosophical perspectives.

Using Bass's own research on genocide and his considerable clinical psychoanalytic experience, the book examines what it is within us that leads us to see some people or groups as "other," what we project onto these groups, how we can come to dehumanize them, and how mass murder can become a purportedly ethical imperative. Using real-life examples, it explores the question of what genocide says about us individually and collectively, how apparently "normal" people can take part in genocide.

Tackling one of the most important topics of our time, this is key reading for all psychoanalysts and psychotherapists, and for philosophers, social scientists, and psychologists.

Alan Bass, PhD, is a psychoanalyst practicing in New York City and is on the graduate philosophy faculty at the New School for Social Research. He is the author of *Difference and Disavowal: The Trauma of Eros*; *Interpretation and Difference: The Strangeness of Care*; and *Fetishism, Psychoanalysis and Philosophy*, many articles, and the translator of four books by Jacques Derrida.

"Grounded in erudite historical research, Alan Bass' psychoanalytic reflections on genocide pose the haunting question if the predilection for mass violence is a manifestation of human nature. Analyzing the unconscious logic of genocide, he demonstrates with compelling theoretical rigor why we need psychoanalysis to understand that genocide presupposes a fetish for purity and fear of contamination and satisfies an unconscious need. This is an urgent and indispensable book in our era of genocidal violence and the emergence of new forms of racism, deportations, and warfare across the globe."

Gabriele M. Schwab is Distinguished Professor Emerita at the University of California, Irvine, with specializations in Comparative Literature and Anthropology. She received her PhD at the University of Constance in 1976 and a PhD in Psychoanalysis from the New Center for Psychoanalysis in LA in 2009. A recipient of a Guggenheim Fellowship and a Heisenberg Fellowship, her work ranges across critical theory, psychoanalysis, trauma studies, ecology, anthropology, and 20th- and 21st-century comparative literatures.

"Alan Bass' book has provided us with a valuable tool for comprehending the incomprehensible "banality of genocide". Drawing on a sophisticated psychoanalytic and philosophical knowledge, he offers a subtle analysis of what is the most hyperbolic implementation of human cruelty."

Sergio Benvenuto, psychoanalyst and philosopher, has been a member of the Italian Council of Scientific Research (Rome). He founded and edited the *European Journal of Psychoanalysis*, and he is the president of Elvio Fachinelli Institute in Italy. He has authored several books in different languages; his most recent work is *Lacan, Kris and the Psychoanalytic Legacy: The Brain Eater* (Routledge).

The Genocide Principle

Perspectives from Psychoanalysis, the Social Sciences, and Philosophy

Alan Bass

Routledge
Taylor & Francis Group
LONDON AND NEW YORK

Designed cover image: Chloe Bass

First published 2027
by Routledge
4 Park Square, Milton Park, Abingdon, Oxon OX14 4RN

and by Routledge
605 Third Avenue, New York, NY 10158

Routledge is an imprint of the Taylor & Francis Group, an informa business

For Product Safety Concerns and Information please contact our EU representative
GPSR@taylorandfrancis.com. Taylor & Francis Verlag GmbH, Kaufingerstraße 24,
80331 München, Germany.

British Library Cataloguing-in-Publication Data
A catalogue record for this book is available from the British Library

ISBN: 978-1-032-91367-4 (hbk)
ISBN: 978-1-032-91065-9 (pbk)
ISBN: 978-1-003-56287-0 (ebk)

DOI: 10.4324/9781003562870

Typeset in Optima
by Newgen Publishing UK

Contents

Introduction
How I Got Here

I was raised in a largely Jewish housing project in Queens, NY. I was taught about the Holocaust and the history of Jewish persecution in Hebrew school, but anti-semitism was something far away, not part of my actual existence. Even one day finding the family car spray-painted in red with swastikas and "Kill Jews" on it did not affect us very much. The assumption was a teenage prank. But near at hand, and indelibly shocking, were the images of violence against civil rights protestors in the South. The hoses, the dogs, the beatings, the bombs, the Klan, and the pure hatred on the faces of white students as Black students attempted to enter their schools. I could not understand it. And I could not understand that the language of my everyday environment, in a largely Jewish, liberal world, tended to be as racist as anything one might hear in the South. Not at home, fortunately. But it was tacitly accepted that there was no point in saying anything about it.

As I entered adolescence, my friends were largely those who were politically minded. We joined civil rights and anti-apartheid demonstrations. And then came college and the anti-war movement. Especially significant was the day that Martin Luther King finally came out against the war, underlining the common logic of the two movements.

Then, in college, partly in Paris, came my discovery of the works of Derrida (initially in 1969; early days) and the entire project of deconstructing "Western metaphysics." The basic idea was that, at its heart, metaphysics was structured by a thinking of difference that it had to exclude, because it upset all axiomatic assumptions. Difference as the "unthought of metaphysics," in Heidegger's famous phrase. Some of the titles alone tell the story: Heidegger's *Identity and Difference,* Derrida's *Writing and Difference*, and Deleuze's *Difference and Repetition*. And then in graduate school came the immersion in Freud, and the decision to pursue training as an analyst. I have now been a practicing analyst for over 40 years.

The everyday clinical work of an analyst is with individuals. As a friend and colleague once put it, there is a world inside of everyone. To effect clinical change is to unearth that world in all its complexity, and then to attempt to modify its structure—an enormous undertaking. But was there any

DOI: 10.4324/9781003562870-1

connection between the deconstruction of metaphysics and clinical work? This was a question I was often asked, and which I inevitably asked myself. The answer came slowly. It was first through a theoretical reconsideration of Freud on the topic of fetishism. The theory of fetishism is supposed to explain how the mind can simultaneously know and not know the same thing about *reality*. I am deliberately emphasizing "reality," because Freud commits a logical fallacy, insistently speaking of sexual difference in terms of "the reality of castration," his insistence that women are *really* castrated. The great surprise, though, is that at the end of his life Freud was also reconsidering his most fundamental ideas about defensive process, starting from the same question: how does the mind simultaneously know and not know the same thing about reality? He came to see that the structure of fetishism was the best illustration of this process. But how to accommodate that insight with the logical fallacy on which the theory is based? This became possible with the realization that, without knowing it, the reality disavowed—known and not known—in fetishism is *the reality of (sexual) difference itself.* But if fetishism is also the model of defensive process, can one go further and assert that there is a fundamentally defensive reaction to difference itself? Why would this be so from a psychoanalytic point of view?

The answers are multiple. They start from the nature of difference. Difference itself is about being *at once* connected to, and separate from, something other. This is the paradox at the heart of fetishism. The mind recoils from simultaneous connection to, and separation from, otherness, and replaces it with fantasies of essential opposites—binary oppositions. (In fetishism this is the opposition phallic/castrated.) But as in metaphysics, the existence of such binary oppositions is based on the exclusion of the difference that structures them. This was not Freud's thought. But he had already begun to see that there is a tendency to narcissistic rejection of difference, the "narcissism of small differences."[1] He had understood that internalization of what he called "fresh *vital* differences" is unconsciously experienced as raising tension levels in the mind, inevitably met by the counteracting tendency to reduce tension levels—in a word, life against death (1920). Clinically, this theory is necessary to understand the manifestations of knowing and not knowing reality—to varying extents, a phenomenon found in everyone. But none of this is integrated in Freud's writings. I have attempted this integration in my previous work.

But my personal deep concern with racism never left me. When I was invited to contribute an essay on racism for a psychoanalytic volume on all forms of prejudice called *Hating in the First Person Plural*, I welcomed the opportunity. Titled *Historical and Unconscious Trauma: Psychoanalysis and Racism*, my essay used clinical material from two patients, one a young man of color and the other a daughter of two Holocaust survivors. Both patients' serious neuroses could not be understood without integrating their individual dynamics with the histories of persecution embedded in their families. Some years later, the editors of that volume, Donald Moss and Lynne Zeavin, were planning a follow-up volume, titled *Hating, Abhorring, and Attempting to Destroy* (from a phrase in Freud's "Instincts and Their Vicissitudes). I was asked if I could contribute another essay on racism. I was initially hesitant. I did not think I had anything new to say. And then Moss wondered whether I would write about Dylann Roof, the young man who had deliberately murdered nine people in a famous Black church in Charleston, South Carolina in 2015.

The murder was all that I knew about Roof. When I started to do research about him, I found that he was preoccupied with the idea that the Black race was an inherent threat to the white race. Race war was necessary for the white race to protect itself against extinction. He wanted his deliberately planned murders to instigate such a war. He had also planned to kill himself immediately after the murder, but did not. He had no remorse about what he had done, claiming that he had purposely chosen what he knew to be "good people," in order to show the necessity of war against all Black people.

There was no question about his guilt, and South Carolina is a death penalty state. His attorney, David Bruck, a known opponent of the death penalty, wanted to save him via an insanity defense, and called expert witnesses to that effect. The prosecution presented expert witnesses to the opposite effect. Roof himself rejected his attorney's strategy, claiming that he was perfectly sane and knew exactly what he was doing and why. He dismissed Bruck, claiming the right to represent himself at his sentencing hearing.

Another hearing was required to determine whether Roof's request was itself due to insanity. The judge finally had to grant him the right to defend himself. When it came time for Roof to speak in his own defense, he was silent. Perhaps the most compelling testimony at this hearing came from the priest who had visited him many times in jail. The priest said that he was utterly confounded by his contact with Roof. On the one hand, he repeatedly told Roof that what he had done was "heinous." On the other hand, he could not reconcile the young man he visited with such actions (Bass, 2021).

The question that faced me was how to write about this. Should I attempt to think about Roof as the troubled young man he clearly was, and how his problems led him to racist murder, the so-called lone shooter phenomenon? Or should I look at him from the point of view of what he claimed he was—a proponent of genocide? I opted for the latter.[2] Having at that point not delved into the genocide literature, I tried to see if I could elaborate something about racist murder itself from a psychoanalytic point of view. Here, all my previous work on disavowal of difference was useful, including Freud's *Group Psychology and the Analysis of the Ego*. In an unusual passage, Freud wrote about a primally violent response to racial difference that he said he could not explain. Again in a nutshell, I used all my prior thinking, along with the work of Narendra Keval on the psychoanalytic understanding of racism, and concepts from Klein and Bion, to explain Roof's actions as the paradoxical combination of normality and psychosis that is at the heart of racial murder. And I brought in Derrida on the questions of undecidability, i.e. the irreducibility of certain paradoxes such that they coexist, e.g. normality and psychosis;

and on the death penalty, which is such a central question in understanding Roof as an exemplar of murderous racism (Bass, 2021).

I had stumbled into the whole question of genocide. As I began to do research on it, it became clear that I did not know the most fundamental, most unwelcome fact about it: at all times and in all places, in the entire history of *Homo sapiens,* there has been genocide. The 1948 UN Convention Against Genocide states that "at all periods of history genocide has inflicted great losses upon humanity" (Preamble, n.p.). It is as intrinsic to humanity as so many other things, for better and for worse. And I had stumbled into one of the questions that much of the vast genocide literature considers: how can normal people do this? Again and again, one finds scholars puzzling over this phenomenon. The overwhelming evidence is that the madness of genocide is committed by people not conventionally "diagnosable," the undecidable question that came up about Roof. As Omer Bartov put it in his *Anatomy of a Genocide*, during the Nazi occupation of one town in Ukraine, the town itself became "an island of normality floating on an ocean of blood" (2018, p. 220). If psychoanalysis is a theory of the unconscious processes intrinsic to the human mind, and if genocide is universal, then it calls for psychoanalytic explanation. Perhaps everything I have said so far is contained in the title of an edited volume on genocide: *Annihilating Difference.*[3]

Having read some major parts of the genocide literature, in the spring of 2023, I taught a course called "Thinking Genocide" in the graduate philosophy department of the New School for Social Research. Some of the participants in the course urged me to make it into a book. That book follows here. I consider it a kind of extended course. For method, I have taken inspiration from the opening chapters of *Group Psychology and the Analysis of the Ego*. There, Freud quoted extensively from such non-psychoanalytic thinkers as Le Bon and McDougall, demonstrating where their ideas on group (or really "crowd," *Masse*) psychology called for integration with psychoanalysis. I will proceed similarly. Each chapter explicates an essential contribution to understanding genocide, and then integrates it with psychoanalytic thought or extends its use of psychoanalytic concepts. As a kind of course, I will try to demonstrate connections between chapters and thinkers, in both text and footnotes. For this purpose there will be necessary repetition of basic points throughout.

Ultimately, it would be immoral to write about genocide simply as an object of study. Can genocide be prevented if it is a pathology intrinsic to the human mind? One genocide scholar, Israel Charny, calls it the "human cancer," a pathology as intrinsic to us as cancer itself. Can cancer be prevented? The post-Holocaust slogan of "never again" has, of course, shown itself to be delusional (Cambodia, Rwanda, etc.), the delusion that genocide is exceptional. To prevent or to treat an illness, one has to know what it is. This has to include confrontation with why it might be nonpreventable or incurable. While this can seem a counsel of despair, the hope is that the greater the knowledge, the greater the chance of discovering where there might be effective intervention. The incurable diseases demand the most prolonged and detailed study.

An Evolutionary Perspective on Genocide

As an introduction, I will begin with Jared Diamond's popular science book, *The Third Chimpanzee: The Evolution and Future of the Human Animal.* Diamond's title is based on the fact that humans share 98.4% of their DNA with two classes of chimps (common and pygmy). His overall project is to trace the evolution of what he considers to be essential human traits—language, art, drugs ... and genocide. Because he knows that genocide is transcultural and transhistorical, and because he is writing for a general audience, the facts he marshals, and the conclusions he comes to, are a means to outline some of the wide questions about genocide, and then to begin to show where psychoanalytic concepts can deepen the analysis. Moreover, genocide as a product of evolution is a question that will be raised in several chapters of this book.

Diamond says that two things jeopardize human existence: our propensity to kill each other and our propensity to destroy our environment (1993, p. 3). While it is obvious that destruction of our environment would jeopardize our existence, why should the propensity to kill each other also do so? This is one of the most important questions about genocide. It immediately suggests the paradox that if genocide might threaten human existence in general, then it is suicidal for the species. How destruction of others might also be self-destruction is a question for which psychoanalysis has a unique answer: according to Freud we have an inherently self-destructive drive that inevitably becomes an other destructive drive, the death drive (Freud, 1920).

Diamond knows that we tend to be uncomfortable thinking of genocide as a basic human trait, and would prefer to see it as a "pathological aberration" (p. 138). Genocide, he says, "is such a painful subject that either we'd rather not think about it at all, or else we'd like to believe that nice people don't commit genocide, only Nazis do ... Are genocidal killers abnormal individuals, or are they normal people?" (p. 277). There are countless observations that people can participate in mass murder, sometimes even enjoy it, and then return to the most ordinary everyday life. Can genocidal killers be both normal and abnormal? Is that possible? Could such "normal abnormality" be a feature of the human mind? This was the question about Roof. There are important psychoanalytic answers to this question too, especially about the coexistence of psychotic and nonpsychotic elements in the mind.

Diamond addresses another crucial paradox about genocide. Humans have developed ethical codes (p. 98). It would seem self-evident that genocide would conflict with the most basic ethical principles. Yet throughout history, killers have "reconciled genocide with their ethical codes" (p. 278). *Ethical* mass murder of innocent victims? How could such a perversion of morality be possible? Psychoanalysis has important things to say about the complex mental mechanisms that can account for this, about how morality itself can be close to cruelty, sadism, destruction, and self-destruction (Freud, 1923).

How might all of this be related to our status as "the third chimpanzee"? Diamond's answer is "chimp xenophobia" (p. 220). The chimps from which we descend massacre each other. He cites Jane Goodall's documented observations of the extermination of one chimpanzee band by another between 1974 and 1977 (p. 291). Chimp genocide is "inefficient"; lacking weapons, they have to kill one at a time (p. 293). Nevertheless, chimps "share xenophobia with us: they clearly recognize members of other bands as different from members of their own band, and treat them very differently…" (p. 294). "Genocidal chimps show intent and planning, however rudimentary" (p. 294).

> of all our human hallmarks […] the one that has been derived most straightforwardly from animal precursors is genocide. Common chimps already carried out planned killings, extermination of neighboring bands, wars of territorial conquest, and abduction of young nubile females.
>
> (p. 294)[4]

Diamond gives compelling anecdotal evidence about intrinsic human xenophobia. He spent many years among the indigenous inhabitants of New Guinea. "As I walked between New Guinea valleys, people who themselves practiced cannibalism and were only a decade out of the Stone Age, routinely warned me about the unspeakably primitive, vile, and cannibalistic habits of the people I would encounter in the next valley" (p. 298). He makes the simple observation that:

> humans practice a dual standard of behavior: strong inhibitions about killing one of "us," but a green light to kill "them" when it was safe to do so. Genocide was acceptable under this dichotomy as an inherited animal instinct or as a uniquely human ethical code
>
> (p. 299)

Perhaps one word of this sentence should be changed: "or." Does not human "us"–"them" dichotomizing, our xenophobic inheritance, compel one to think "and"? That humans have developed an ethical code out of "animal instinct"? This is part of standard psychoanalytic theory. The ethical part of us, the "super-ego," is in direct relation to our "instincts," including our most violent ones (Freud, 1923). While we tend to think of this only in terms of suppression, or repression, of instincts, if "they" represent something intolerable or threatening to "us," we can channel those instincts into ethically justified murder of "them." Diamond summarizes: "…we, like so many modern people, reconciled genocide with a universal code of ethics. The solution was to plead self-defense and overriding principle, and to view the victims as savage animals" (p. 300). Does dichotomizing xenophobia alone explain how genocide can be justified as self-defense, and how evidently human victims can be viewed as non-human, beastly? Might this, again, be related to the coexistence of psychotic and non-psychotic elements in the mind? The *belief* that other humans are not human, are beasts, parasites, germs, such that it becomes ethically justified to kill them, is strictly speaking a delusion. A delusion that at very least suggests the psychoanalytic concept of projection. "Our" murderousness is justified, because "they" are the murderous enemy. This is a theme examined throughout this volume.

Diamond lists four typical motives for genocide: (1) A militarily stronger people attempts to occupy the land of a weaker people who resist; (2) power struggles within a pluralistic society, leading one group to kill the other group: (3) scapegoat killings of a helpless minority; and (4) racial and religious persecution. Racial and religious motives, however, are actually the most general and contribute to the other three (p. 289).

Diamond provides world maps and charts illustrating what he labels "Some Genocides, 1492-1900; Some Genocides, 1900-1950; and Some Genocides, 1950-1990" (pp. 284–6). I take his "some" to be both factual and ironic. It suggests that it would probably be impossible to schematize "all," which is precisely the question of this book.

Notes

1 In the chapter on Bauman (Chapter 2), we will see that Freud introduced the "narcissism of minor differences" via the primal experience of sexual difference as something strange, uncanny, and threatening. This could have been the corrective to the "reality of castration." The strange *reality of difference* defensively becomes the "reality of castration," which of course makes the woman a version of the man, eliminating sexual difference.

2 Eventually I found this decision justified in an article on the many legal disputes about what constitutes crimes against humanity and genocide. "Thus, at least theoretically, an individual acting alone, without any state involvement, may still perpetrate the crime of genocide, provided that he or she intends to destroy a protected group in whole or in part" (Schabas, p. 98).

3 I will return to this volume in my conclusion.

4 A study not cited by Diamond, "Lethal coalitionary attacks of chimpanzees (*Pan troglodytes troglodytes* on gorillas (*Gorilla, gorilla, gorilla*) in the wild" (L. Southern, T. Deschner, S. Pika) documents carefully observed attacks by a band of chimps on gorillas, which included eating a baby gorilla. The authors conclude:

> Ultimately, additional observations in combination with isochronous assessments of fruit availability and dietary overlap are needed to differentiate whether coalitionary attacks are indeed the output of interspecific predation spurred by opportunistic hunting, interspecies competition for food resources or whether these interactions are merely a non-adaptive by-product of the 'xenophobic nature' of chimpanzees.
>
> (n.p.)

The authors' resistance to the idea of chimp xenophobia is contained in the words "merely" and "nonadaptive." However, the possibility that chimp xenophobia could be nonadaptive also suggests that it might not be to their evolutionary advantage.

1 History

Ben Kiernan's *Blood and Soil: A World History of Genocide from Sparta to Darfur* is a magisterial work. Kiernan, a historian, started as an expert on the Cambodian genocide. *Blood and Soil*—from the Nazi slogan—was published in 2007, winning several awards. Kiernan provides exceptional detail about the world history of genocide, much of which is startling and invaluable. Given this wide historical knowledge, Kiernan's generalizations about genocide are compelling. I will use his work to extend the introduction of psychoanalytic thinking.

Kiernan's first generalization is that "Genocidal thinking usually involves idealized conceptions of the world, utopian or dystopian, divorced from reality but capable of being forcefully imposed upon it" (p. 21). This is already complex. What does "thinking" mean here? The simple answer, the one probably intended, is: how do people claim that genocide is necessary, or justified? From the psychoanalytic point of view, however, this is not sufficient. Thinking for Freud is "secondary process," conscious, rational thought. It is made possible by the capacity to delay gratification, to tolerate tension without immediately discharging it—primary process. Freud calls secondary process the "reality principle," as opposed to the primary process "pleasure principle" (1911). It is basic to psychoanalysis that "thinking," secondary process, the reality principle, can be usurped by the pleasure principle. We might want to believe that we are making rational decisions, when in fact we are rationalizing our wishes for immediate gratification. In genocide, we can even believe that we are making an ethical decision, as Diamond put it in his juxtaposition of animal instinct and ethics. This is nowhere better illustrated than in Heinrich Himmler's statement that "We had the moral right, we had the duty to our people, to destroy this people [the Jews] which wanted to destroy us" (cited by Kiernan, p. 452). Here, we have an example of delusion, as also mentioned in our discussion of Diamond. It is taken as fact that the Jews wanted to destroy the Germans. Once this is so, it is only rational and moral to protect "our people." This sounds like "thinking." But it clearly serves the need to discharge tension—whatever that tension might be—, the usurpation of the reality principle by the pleasure principle.

DOI: 10.4324/9781003562870-2

Kiernan has said that this "thinking" involves "idealized conceptions of the world." "Idealized" suggests "not real," "too perfect." From the psychoanalytic point of view, this suggests two things: fantasy and narcissism. "Of the world," "divorced from reality," "capable of being forcefully imposed upon it," suggest that such narcissistic fantasies are all encompassing; they are a *compulsion* to explain the world. That they are divorced from reality again suggests delusion—psychosis. That they are capable of being forcefully imposed upon the world and reality suggests that they do have a kind of skewed rationality; otherwise, they could not be imposed upon the world. But this requires *force*. Where does this force come from?

The obvious answer is aggression. Idealized conceptions of the world are aggressively *forced* upon reality and the world. Reality and the world, here, means people: a delusional, narcissistic fantasy is "forcefully imposed" on a specific group. That such delusions can be *forced* upon one's own group of people (e.g., compelling the Germans to believe that the Jews wanted to destroy them) implies that there is receptivity to such "thinking"; otherwise, the *force* would be useless. In other words, at least some of one's group already harbors such "thoughts" (narcissistic fantasies, idealizations). Hence, those group members are *ready* to believe that they are threatened by an external force (e.g., the Jews), such that the (forceful) imposition of genocidal delusion is rational and ethical.

Kiernan then analyzes the frequent role of racism in genocide:

> Racism is an ideology, an idealist concept lacking material basis [...] Prejudice promoting genocide may thus arise from suppositions of a victim group's innate *inferiority* (in a static view of history) or its historical anteriority (in a progressive view) or even from a perceived threat of domination by a group possessing alleged *superiority* [...] racism is often accompanied by dominating ambition. Usually expressed as a phobia of contamination, political racism also disguises a forceful demand on all members of one's own group to maintain distance from another group
>
> (p. 22)

Again, Kiernan starts with "idealist," without "material basis," i.e., fantasy-based. Such fantasies may be assumptions of "inferiority," related to a "static view of history." In other words, "they" have always been, and always will be, like this—inferior, worthless, subhuman. Such a "static view of history" assumes timelessness, something that cannot be altered by time. "Timelessness," for Freud, is characteristic of the unconscious. Just as dreams have only one temporal mode, the present, unconscious processes in general exist in a permanent now. What Kiernan calls the "progressive view" is related to "historical anteriority," i.e., a temporal movement from then to now. This implies the conscious relation to time, in which there is past, present, and future. But note that this historicization takes its point of departure from fantasy. The inferior group may have been there before us, but "we" have changed since then. Even so, there might always be a threat to "our" existence. "They" might change too, and become a stronger, superior group. It only makes sense to eliminate such a threat. Thus, one way or another "racism is often accompanied by dominating ambition" related to fantasies of inferiority or superiority. Psychoanalytically this is the typical "all or nothing" mode of narcissistic thought. Either "they" are worthless or "they" possess an almost omnipotent power. How are "we" to dominate "them"? The answer is by obtaining *omnipotent* control over them which is another crucial aspect of narcissism.

Kiernan says that this "dominating ambition" is usually expressed as a "phobia of contamination." Whether inferior or superior "they" possess the insidious power to get inside us, and to ruin us. When Kiernan calls this "phobia," I assume he means "phobia" in the usual sense of an irrational fear, a fear of being destroyed from the inside. To quell the fear of contamination is to prevent the possibility of "their" getting inside. Given their power to contaminate, as Kiernan says, the only option is to stay away, to avoid contact. This suggests the defense mechanism of "splitting." But if splitting is not absolute, then the threat of contamination itself has to be eliminated by extermination.

What if one took Kiernan's word "phobia" in its more psychoanalytic sense? Certainly, phobias are irrational fears. But they have a complex structure. From Freud's point of view, in a phobia, whatever one is apparently afraid of is not what one is really afraid of. There has been a displacement from one fear to another. For example, a childhood fear of animals can be a displacement of the fear of punishment from the oedipal parent onto the animal. A fear of open spaces may be a fear of sexual temptation. Would this logic deepen Kiernan's point? What displacement might have occurred in the racist fear that "they" can "contaminate" us, such that "we" have to stay away at all cost? Perhaps that "we" cannot stay away. Perhaps we ultimately do not have the absolute boundary that would prevent them from ruining us from the inside. In a sense, we are "porous." "They" can always get inside us; they are a "virus." Hitler said that the discovery of the "Jewish virus" was one of the great achievements of science, on a par with the discoveries of Koch and Pasteur.[1] Moreover, they can get inside "us" sexually, reproducing more of them. Hence, all the laws against, or extreme condemnation of, miscegenation.

Kiernan then refers this phobic structure to one's "group." This opens up all the issues of group psychology. One knows what kinds of forceful demands to stay away from the contaminating group he means: the various forms of segregation, forced migration, internment, and death. If all of "us" stay away from all of "them," or ultimately if they are eliminated, "they" will not infect us. Strength in numbers will counteract our essential porousness. The "body politic" will be immunized. But until the body politic is immunized, while the threat of contamination is "real," "social distancing" is necessary. "We" have to maintain distance from "them," precisely because we are ultimately porous.

To understand this psychoanalytically, we need to say more about splitting. The basic idea is that two opposed fantasies—good/bad, superior/inferior—have to be kept apart emotionally so that the one does not "infect" the other. One has to "know" that these categories are unconditionally opposed. But if "we" might always be "infected" by them, we must double and re-double our efforts to convince ourselves that we are dealing with an unconditional opposition, an opposition of essences. "They" are categorically harmful, no matter how harmless they might *appear.* In fact, should they *appear* to be just like us, we must not be deluded. Recall Diamond's New Guineans for whom people in the next valley were irredeemably evil, although ethnically identical. The mountains separating the valleys are the geographical image of splitting.

Kiernan then expands his analysis:

> Scientific racism incorporates parables about ancient human bloodlines, breeding, and pest extermination [...] Genocidal intent requires a predilection for massive violence and the targeting of an unarmed or relatively poorly armed victim group. That mindset usually comes with an expansionist territorial drive, bolstered by a sense of historical loss and racial or religious resentment. Those notions in turn connect to concepts of superior and inferior occupants. As idealist predilections, there is much in common between racism or religious prejudice and notions of biological purity, historical decline, and rural romanticism
>
> (p. 27)

The incorporation of parable into science again illustrates the way that allegedly logical thought is actually a form of fantasy. Again, the fantasies of what can get inside us, infecting our blood, our race, via infectious agents. But now Kiernan speaks of a "predilection for massive violence." "Predilection" implies a disposition, or even desire. Given the universality of genocide, is such a predilection a manifestation of human nature? The passage on the violent response to racial difference in Freud's *Group Psychology and the Analysis of the Ego* (mentioned in our introduction, "How I Got Here"), is about the same topic. Like Kiernan here, it addresses an indisputable fact, but is admittedly vague. Freud speaks of the human "predilection" (to use Kiernan's word) for racial prejudice, and says that "it is unmistakable that in this whole connection men give evidence of a readiness for hatred, an aggressiveness, the source of which is unknown, and to which one is tempted to ascribe an elementary character" (1920, 100–101). "Unknown source," "elementary character": something primal and inexplicable that leads to hatred and aggression.

In 1920, Freud published *Beyond the Pleasure Principle.* He footnotes a reference to it (1920, p. 101), but does not link the "elementary character" of racial hatred to the death drive. This seems essential to me. His idea that a self-destructive drive is inevitably projected onto others as the source of human aggression means that we *must* destroy others in order not to destroy ourselves. Would this not be one aspect of the explanation of the predilection for massive violence against the racial other? And would this not imply that self and other destructiveness are inextricably intertwined?

Kiernan makes two important observations about the pragmatics of genocide. "Genocidal enterprises, ambitious by definition, require an ideological inflexibility so severe that, ironically, pragmatic skill is required to implement them" (p. 33). "The challenge of predicting and then preventing genocide is to identify in advance the obsessions that drive domination and violence and the ideological predilections that overrule their own inherent tensions and pragmatic impossibilities" (p. 35).

"Ideological inflexibility" again suggests the unshakeable conviction that a delusion is true ("the Jews want to destroy us"). But to protect "ourselves" against destruction is a massive undertaking, requiring mobilization of all our resources. "We" *must* maintain our certainty that this is possible; otherwise, "we" will be subject to the unbearable "tension" that this is simply, "pragmatically" impossible. It suggests that our "ideological inflexibility" is in fact a rigid defense against what we really know, and are haunted by, (as Kiernan says): the inherent tension that the task is pragmatically impossible. This is akin to the phobia of contamination, which obscures our knowledge that despite "our" best efforts, "we" are porous, open to contamination.

In a small paper of 1924 Freud had analyzed the structure of delusions. There he said that delusions are a "patch" over a lost piece of reality, an unbearable piece of reality (1924a, p. 151). The maintenance of the delusional patch requires that the

> ego creates, autocratically, a new external and internal world; and there can be no doubt of two facts—that this new world is constructed in accordance with the id's wishful impulses, and that the motive of this dissociation from the external world is some very serious frustration by reality of a wish—a frustration which seems intolerable
>
> (1924a, p. 151)

Recall Kiernan on "idealized conceptions of the world ... divorced from reality but capable of being forcefully imposed upon it." He has observed what Freud analyzes here. Genocidal "thinking" is a clear example of usurpation of the reality principle (secondary process, delay of discharge), by the pleasure principle (wishful discharge of tension).

This "thinking" serves to maintain the conviction that the unbearable tension of porousness, of the pragmatic impossibility of the genocidal project, can be "wished away" by the "forceful imposition" of a narcissistically idealized, "autocratically" created "new external and internal world." This is a "world" in which "we" can eliminate the unbearable so that "we" are no longer disturbed by it. Extending this logic in *The Loss of Reality in Neurosis and Psychosis* (1924b), Freud said that:

> In a psychosis, the transforming of reality is carried out upon the psychical precipitates of former relations to it—that is, upon the memory-traces, ideas and judgements which have been previously derived from reality and by which reality was represented in the mind [...] Thus, the psychosis is also faced with the task of procuring for itself perceptions of a kind which shall correspond to the new reality; and this is most radically effected by means of hallucination
>
> (1924b, pp. 185, 186)

The other way is by means of forceful imposition of delusion. The paradox here, is that once the world is so reconstructed, all the "pragmatic skills" that the reality principle demands are maintained. Hence, the seemingly realistic, nonpsychotic implementation of the genocidal project, in whatever form it takes:[2] The coexistence of normality and psychosis. Whether one is dealing with a "lone shooter" (like Dylann Roof) or an entire government carrying out genocide, if one is to predict and possibly prevent genocide, one has to understand an elementary principle of psychosis: one cannot argue with a delusion. It is the "truth," and logically consistent once a "new internal and external world" has been created in conformity with the "patch" over the unbearable reality.

Here one encounters the terrible reality of the unpreventable and the incurable.

To illustrate this, and to extend the analysis further, let us turn to Kiernan on the Cambodian genocide, for which he has special expertise. The roots of the Cambodian genocide are in fanatical prejudice against their neighbors, the Vietnamese:

> As early as 1750, Western missionaries reported that by order of the Khmer king, '[t]he Cambodians have massacred all the Cochinese [Vietnamese] they could find in the country.' For six weeks, 'this order was executed very precisely and very cruelly,' and no survivors were found.
>
> (p. 548)

"In April 1970, the French ambassador to Phnom Penh warned that new massacres of thousands of ethnic Vietnamese by the pro-American forces of Lon Nol's Khmer Republic could become 'real genocide'" (p. 548). In 1978 Pol Pot promoted national and class hatred for the Vietnamese enemy, to materialize it:

> In his view, an idea became concrete by bloodshed [...] the CPK [Khmer Communist Party] leadership employed biological metaphors that suggest the threat of contamination. It referred to enemies as 'diseased elements,' 'microbes,' 'pests buried within,' and traitors 'boring in,' just as the Nazis had talked of Jews as 'vermin' and 'lice.'
>
> (p. 549)

To make concrete the idea that contaminating elements have to be eliminated by bloodshed is precisely the process of confirming the reality of a delusionally created external world. The actual sight of blood vindicates the idea, i.e., fantasy, that the infectious agent is being cleansed. "As this fetish for purity suggests, despite the CPK's Marxist–Leninist heritage, its ideology was antimaterialist, again resembling racialist thinking elsewhere" (p. 550).

Kiernan's use of the word "fetish," as in his use of "phobia," is meant in the popular sense of compulsive overvaluation, as when one speaks of an extreme sexual overvaluation of a particular material object (e.g., a certain type of shoe). But he has intuitively grasped a basic psychoanalytic point. The fetishist believes that it is the shoe itself that arouses him. But the arousal is the result of the imposition of a fantasy onto the shoe. While the shoe embodies a fantasy for the psychoanalytic observer, its material reality disavows that process. The shoe is experienced concretely, to use Kiernan's word about bloodshed, as concretely as the sight of food would be if I am very hungry. It would be absurd to think that the sight of food when I am hungry *means* anything other than the obvious. Similarly, for the sexual fetishist, the shoe itself has no meaning; it is not symbolic. This is why the logic of fetishism is the explanation of the general problem of what is clinically called "concreteness," as when a patient speaks of something that for the analyst is potentially meaningful, but for the patient is not.[3]

In the introductory remarks, I summarized my work on fetishism as the imposition of two opposed fantasies over a tension-raising difference—simultaneous connection and separation. In Kiernan's discussion of the ideology of the Khmer Rouge, these are the common genocidal fantasies of pure and impure, akin to the common fantasies of superior and inferior. They are imposed over the Cambodians' intolerable connection to, and separation from, the Vietnamese, as in Diamond's example of the indigenous people of New Guinea. However, it is one thing for a sexual fetishist to maintain the belief in the actual power of a material object, but quite another when this logic confirms the necessity of genocide. There is a common denominator: the defense against intolerable difference. But to make genocide mandatory, there is an equally mandatory delusion that one's intact identity depends upon protection against the threat of contamination by the different other. This means that the threat never really goes away, because ultimately that identity is porous. Thus, as Kiernan says, the Khmer Rouge had to turn against its own group. "Soon, even most of the Khmer victims were accused of having 'Khmer bodies with Vietnamese minds'…" (p. 549). "The resulting bloodbath killed over 100,000, possibly as many as 250,000 eastern Khmers, as the CPK internalized its own threat of racial destruction…" (p. 550).[4]

Once more we have to return to Freud on the primally violent response to racial difference, and its relation to the death drive. When Kiernan says that the CPK "internalized its own threat of racial destruction," he is describing events the way a historian does: this happened, and then that happened. The CPK *eventually* turned its threat of racial destruction inward. But from a psychoanalytic point of view, this might be backward. If there is a self-destructive drive that is projected outward onto the destruction of the other, such that self-destruction and other destructions are inextricably intertwined, then the "internalization" of the threat of racial destruction was there from the beginning. Dylann Roof planned to kill himself after his murders, but instead did everything to have the state do it for him. In an extension of this logic, Kiernan describes how the state *necessarily* becomes the executioner of its own people. He summarizes:

> In the case of the Hutu of Rwanda, as with the Khmer majority under DK [Democratic Kampuchea] and even the Germans under Nazism, the subjection of individuals to the overwhelming interest of their 'race' only made them more vulnerable to violence purportedly 'protecting' them from racial contamination
>
> (p. 559)

Purification as self-destruction.[5]

Freud himself uses the word "purified" in a context directly related to this issue. In *Instincts and Their Vicissitudes*, he speaks of the early ego's tendency to project all unpleasure outside itself, such that it becomes a "purified pleasure ego" (1915a, p. 136). Crucially, this is why Freud also says that "hate as a relation to objects is older than love" (1915a). He means that the distinction between self and other can be based on the pleasure principle's automatic tendency to reduce tension. If I feel tension within myself, I project it outward, such that an object outside myself embodies this tension. It is a threat to my self-preservation. Hence, "We feel the 'repulsion' of the object, and hate it; this hate can afterwards be intensified to the point of an aggressive inclination against the object—an intention to destroy it" (1915, p. 137). But it must be emphasized that this is an intention to destroy an object who embodies what has been intolerable within oneself. Freud goes further:

> The ego hates, abhors and pursues with intent to destroy all objects which are a source of unpleasurable feeling for it, *without taking into account* whether they mean a frustration of sexual satisfaction or of *the satisfaction of self-preservative needs*
>
> (1915a, p. 138; my emphasis)

If racial difference itself is an unbearable tension, then I hate the racial "other"; I must destroy it. But such destructiveness does not take into account, does not think about, how this apparent attempt to protect oneself might also be a threat to one's own self-preservation. This it has to be, since I am unconsciously destroying something that comes from me. This is also the logic of the death drive—my self-destructiveness becomes the destruction of the other: purification as self-destruction.

Studying the Rwandan genocide, Kiernan cites documents used by Hutu propagandists to incite genocide against Tutsis. These included explicit encouragement to use the technique called "accusation in the mirror" (p. 569). "Perpetrator regimes appear to sense that if genocide can ever be justified, it is only as a defense against genocide" (p. 569). In a word, accuse your victim of victimizing you. "We" do not have genocidal intent. "They" do, so we have no choice but to respond in kind—another version of "the Jews want to destroy us." This seems to be a simple use of projection. But the structure of accusation in the mirror is more complex. The propagandist already "knows" (delusionally) that the intended victims are actually, concretely, "vermin," a virus. Given what "they" are, "they" have no choice but to want to destroy "us." We have no choice but to act in self-defense.

If one then integrates "accusation in the mirror" with the ideas of the purified pleasure ego's projection of unpleasure and the death drive, one can understand that the projection—"they" are genocidal—would seem to turn back on the accuser, who is *also* unconsciously "looking in the mirror," accusing himself. But again this is so only for an observer, just as for the observer the fetishist's shoe embodies a fantasy. Dylann Roof said that he did not hate Black people, he only hated what they do (Bass, 2021, p. 305)—always commit violence against white people. This is a clear use of accusation in the mirror: Roof himself intended to eliminate Black people. He *also* planned to commit suicide—the intertwining of self and other destruction.

In a law journal article titled *Accusation in the Mirror*, Kenneth Marcus argues for the reasons why even before actual genocide, accusation in the mirror should be considered direct incitement to violence, as in a case like Roof's. But he also recognizes what is "counterintuitive" about it. He summarizes:

> The basic idea of AiM is deceptively simple: propagandists must impute to enemies exactly what they and their own party are planning to do. In other words, AiM is a rhetorical practice in which one falsely accuses one's enemies of conducting, plotting, or desiring to commit precisely the same transgressions that one plans to commit against them [...] This may seem an unlikely means of inciting mass-murder, since it would intuitively seem likely not only to fail but also to backfire by publicly telegraphing its speakers' malicious intentions [...] The counter-intuitiveness of this method is best appreciated when one grasps that its injunctions are to be taken literally. There is no hyperbole in the Note's [found in the Hutu Butare prefecture after the Rwandan genocide] directive that the propagandist should 'impute to enemies exactly what they and their own party are planning to do.' The point is not merely to impute iniquities that are as bad as the misdeeds that the propagandist's own party intends. Instead, AiM is the more audacious idea of charging one's adversary with 'exactly' the misdeeds that the propagandist's party intends to commit
>
> (p. 359)

For the observer, the fetishist's shoe embodies a fantasy; for the fetishist it does not. Analogously, for the observer the genocidal propagandist's "accusation in the mirror" embodies his intent. For the receptive recipient it does not: "its injunctions are to be taken literally," concretely. Marcus is asking how the propagandist can "know," however intuitively, that this will work.

Here we must marshal more psychoanalytic theory, specifically on the nature of projection. It is not well known that in 1922 Freud wrote a small paper, titled *Some Neurotic Mechanisms in Homosexuality, Jealousy and Paranoia*, in which he refined his previous thoughts about projection. The paranoid or jealous person does not simply project "into the blue" (1922, p. 226). Rather, he or she has intuitively grasped something that is *unconsciously* true about the other, even if that other does not consciously behave in conformity with that truth (1922). This may sound like a kind of mind reading, but it is consistent with Freud's thought that it is possible for one unconscious to be receptive to, to "read" another.

Marcus begins to approach this topic in his article, demonstrating the necessity of integrating psychoanalytic theory with genocide scholarship. He says that AiM is "sufficiently commonplace to be readily understood—in its gruesome implications—by its hearers," and that it is "strikingly effective, not only at motivating genocide but also at meeting the perpetrators' psychological needs" (p. 359). In other words, there is a kind of "meeting of the minds" between propagandist and listener. A need is fulfilled in each. This is why Marcus briefly mentions what he calls "an inconvenient insight," namely that "AiM, while sometimes a deliberate propagandistic tactic, also sometimes expresses an unconscious impulse" (p. 372).

Does the "inconvenience" of the insight illustrate both the necessity of, and perhaps resistance to, the necessity of understanding an unconscious process? Marcus relies on projection: "no phenomenon ... better exemplifies the defense mechanism that prejudice, classically, has been understood to provide. 'Projection' is the process of displacing unwanted feelings onto despised others, who may then appear to be external threats" (p. 383). The perpetrator can unconsciously "know" that his need to project will work because he also "knows" that his propaganda will not fall on deaf ears. It will be "readily understood—in its gruesome implications—by its hearers." As in Freud's idea that projection includes intuition of the other's unconscious, the propagandist "knows" that the recipient consciously or unconsciously will be receptive, because the defensive, hateful response to racial difference is operative in everyone. But it must always be kept in mind that on both sides, one is dealing with *the unconscious process of forming a "purified pleasure ego" that is also a manifestation of the death drive*.

This leads to further refinement of the theory of projection via the work of Melanie Klein. A summary is necessary. From the beginning of her work, Klein took Freud's idea that self-destruction is projected onto an external object literally (1975, p. 126). The earliest forms of anxiety are in relation to the death drive; the projection of it is a response to that anxiety. Any frustration that a baby feels, akin to the unpleasurable tensions Freud describes, leads to projection of the death drive onto the frustrating object. This becomes the fantasy of the "bad breast," the original persecutory object. All gratification is then attributed to a "good breast." The good breast is idealized: it is the source of all pleasure. Extreme splitting is necessary: good and bad must not touch, for bad might *contaminate* good. Here we find another explanation of the narcissistic idealization of one's group that must be kept apart from the bad, persecutory group that actually embodies one's own self-destructiveness. Klein calls this the paranoid-schizoid position (1986, p. 177) because it depends upon the mechanisms of projection and splitting. Whether this is a process in the mind of an infant is open to question. That it is a process always potentially available to anyone is not, as the universality of genocide illustrates.

Two further developments of Klein's thinking are necessary. For the psyche to emerge from the unmitigated aggression of the paranoid-schizoid position, splitting has to be overcome. Good and bad have to be integrated, their separation undone. They have to touch. But if they touch, bad could contaminate good; good might be lost. Klein calls this the depressive position, because Freud's theory of depression centers on the idea of object loss. Thus, the depressive position entails its own set of extreme anxieties. If one can deal with these anxieties, it becomes possible to take responsibility for all the aggression of the paranoid-schizoid position. One can experience "the disaster of one's sadism." But if this is not possible, there is inevitable regression to the paranoid-schizoid position (1986, p. 190). Genocide is the paranoid-schizoid position writ large.

In a further extension of her theorizing, Klein, like Freud, refined the theory of projection. Freud spoke of projection of unpleasurable tension *onto* an external object. It was always part of Klein's thinking that there are fantasies of projecting the "badness" from within oneself *into* an external object. In a 1946 paper she said that the projection of one's own "badness" *into* the object creates an identification with the object. She called this "projective identification," and said that it is the model of an aggressive object relation (1986, p. 183). This is another mechanism implicit in "accusation in the mirror." The need to create a "bad," persecutory object in order to defend against one's own self-destructiveness allows one to *believe*, to *know* (delusion), that the impetus to destruction comes from the outside. It is sensible and ethical to defend against it. Members of one's own group need to join this crusade in their own interest. And they can be recruited, because of the implicit aggression against racial difference that Freud spoke of. The need to split "our" goodness from "their" badness prepares the ground. As Marcus adumbrated, unconscious needs are satisfied for both propagandists and recruits. It is as if the propagandist has grasped Freud's point that projection assumes "knowledge" of the other's unconscious. The "goodness" of one's racial identity can be contaminated by the "badness" of the inevitable persecutors. The conviction is that everyone uses the defenses of projective identification and splitting (Klein), which in fact is always potentially the case.

If this is so, then, as Marcus says, the propagandist can be confident that the injunction to genocide will be heard and taken literally, concretely. When it comes to the issue of racial difference, again returning to Freud on primal violence, one does not have to be psychotic to be receptive to the "truth" of a delusional structure.

The question has often been raised of whether everyone is potentially genocidal. Certainly, this is what perpetrators believe. But then one also has to look at why there have always been those who see the madness of genocide, who protest against it. Kiernan gives some striking examples. In the 16th century, the Spanish cleric Bartolome de Las Casas called the conquest of Guatemala and extermination of its indigenous people a "holocaust" (p. 93). In a striking passage on the progressive extermination of the Indians of the American colonies, Benjamin Franklin wrote:

> If an Indian injures me does it follow that I may revenge that Injury on all Indians? It is well known that Indians are of different Tribes, Nations and Languages, as well as White People. In Europe, if the French, who are White People, should injure the Dutch, are they to revenge it on the English, because they too are White People? The only Crime of these poor Wretches seems to have been, that they had a reddish-brown Skin, and black Hair; and some People of that Sort, it seems had murdered some of our Relations. If it be right to kill Men for such a Reason, then should any Man, with a freckled Face and red Hair kill a Wife or Child of mine, it would be right for me to revenge it, by killing *all* the freckled and red-haired Men, Women, and Children
>
> (cited, p. 246; my emphasis)

The first genocide of the 20th century, not sufficiently known, was the destruction of the Herero people of Southwest Africa by Germany. "August Bebel called the destruction of the Herero not just barbaric, but bestial. Bebel accepted neither racial hierarchy nor racial purity, and he even ridiculed German fears of 'mixed races'" (p. 387). To reject racial hierarchy and purity (Bebel), to see the absurdity of racist revenge (Franklin), to label one's country's actions a "holocaust" (de Las Casas), is not to employ the defenses of the paranoid-schizoid position: projective identification and splitting. It is to have maintained the depressive position. It is to see into delusion, to be able to resist the usurpation of secondary process by primary process. It is to see the "disaster created by one's own sadism."

Another crucial, and again startling, aspect of the history of "genocidal thinking" discerned by Kiernan is the role of the Bible. It is well known that the Old Testament god proscribed murder (the Sixth Commandment) but prescribed capital punishment. Less well known, perhaps, is the precise description of genocide in Numbers 31:1-19. Yahweh orders Moses to exact vengeance on the Midianites. Not only were the Midianite kings, allies, and men to be killed, but also all the male children, and all the women who were not virgins. The girls were to be allotted to the Israelites, the towns burned, and all livestock taken as bounty. In other words, complete elimination of the Midianites. Genocide. Another example is the Amalekites. In Deuteronomy 25:16–18, the Israelites had been commanded to completely destroy the inhabitants of idolatrous cities in Canaan, along with their livestock. Deuteronomy 25:17–19 recounts the command to completely expunge the memory of Amalek, to eliminate them as if they had never existed. In 1 Samuel 15:1–9 Saul is again commanded to destroy the Amalekites, killing men, women, children, and babies.[6]

In the Biblical accounts the Midianites and the Amalekites were guilty of crimes against the Israelites and of idolatry. The command to take vengeance on *all* of them, men, women, and children, is a version of the genocidal logic so well limned by Franklin: their guilt is "racialized." How can this square with the commandment not to kill? That commandment must be understood in two ways, legalistic and xenophobic. We are not to kill each other, *except* if we commit certain crimes: the legality of capital punishment. And while we are not to kill each other, it is justified to kill our enemies, especially those who (in psychoanalytic terms) are bad, persecutory objects. Unconscious logic will have it that there will always be such objects (racial difference). Since they might always grow stronger, posing a genocidal threat against "us," we must gain *omnipotent* control over the threat. That control is enjoined upon us by an omnipotent, sovereign power: in the Bible, the one, true God. Ethics and instinct, as Diamond described, are then one and the same. The unconscious logic of genocide found in the Bible is another instance of its universality.

Christian Europeans could then take inspiration and justification for genocidal actions from the Biblical accounts. During his long war against the Saxons:

> Charlemagne had 4,500 Saxon prisoners 'beheaded in a single day,' according to the Royal Frankish Annals. Posing as Israelites in a new promised land, Charlemagne's army had apparently drawn inspiration from the biblical massacres of the Amalekites and Moabites [*sic*; this might be a mistake; Midianites would be more accurate]
>
> (p. 64)

Sepulveda, a Spanish rhetorician, said that "'for their sins ... inhabitants of the Promised Land were exterminated by the Children of Israel.' Yet Sepulveda also condemned the Jews, whose 'extermination God desired because of their crimes and idolatry'" (p 75). During the long extermination of the Indians of North America, the question of its justification was sometimes asked. Kiernan cites one English colonist's words: "Should not Christians have more mercy and compassion? ... Sometimes the Scripture declareth women and children must perish with their parents ... We had sufficient light from the Word of God for our proceedings" (p. 231).

The great irony of history is that Germany took inspiration for genocide from the American precedent. Supporting the Americans' sometimes biblically justified destruction of the Indians, Thomas Jefferson said that "The confined brutalization, if not extermination of this race in America is therefore to form an added chapter in English history of the same colored man in Asia" (cited, p. 329). When August Bebel in Germany denounced the slaughter of the Hereros, "...there were objections to such criticisms, supported by the American precedent to exterminate the Indians. Past genocides provided both precedent and excuse for current ones" (p. 387). Dernberg, an apologist for the genocide of the Herero, said that in the course of civilization some native tribes, like some animals, must be destroyed if they are not to become degenerate. He cited the United States as the greatest example of colonization the world had known, beginning with the almost total annihilation of the original inhabitants (p. 388).

The important implication of the through line from the Bible to America to Germany is that the logic of genocide is underpinned by the idea of sovereign power, whether of a god or the state. French psychoanalyst Rene Major adds an important insight on this question: "...the mythical violence that attempts to found the right to a new order needs to depend upon divine violence to establish the justice of its cause, a violence irreducible to law, a violence that destroys law" (1999, p. 142). Once there is divinity, there is omnipotence: gods have greater than human power. Their "law" is greater than human law. Hence, they provide justification for the amalgamation of law and ethics with mass murder. Kiernan provides explicit examples of how this could work. To justify territorial expansion, "Colonists applied the legal terms *vacuum domicilium* in North America and *terra nullis* in Australia, divesting the indigenous inhabitants not only of land ownership, but sometimes even of their presence" (p. 165). He adds that the exterminations that accompany territorial expansion are underwritten by "murderous hatred" (p. 168).

In a closing statement to his book, Kiernan reiterates his themes that "...fetishes of purity and contamination have strengthened the racism and violence that promote genocide" (p. 606). Hence, "The cure and prevention of the crime of genocide must lie at least in part in the diagnosis of its recurring causes and symptoms" (p. 606). Cure and prevention depend upon the "inconvenient insight" that genocide depends upon unconscious processes. Fetishes of purity and contamination are symptomatic of the relation between fetishism itself and the paranoid-schizoid position. Fetishism is the defense against intolerable difference. In genocide this is primarily racial difference, which is both narcissistically intolerable and ineliminable, provoking the primal self and other destructiveness of the death drive. In response to the tensions of the intolerable and the ineliminable, racial difference becomes the delusional fantasy of contamination and purification. This is the "diagnosis" of genocide's "recurring causes and symptoms."

Notes

1 See Königsberg, *Ideology, Perception, and Genocide: How Fantasy Generates History* (n.d.):

> The image of Jew as virus or bacteria was present in the minds of leading Nazis as the killing process unfolded in 1942 and 1943. In February 1942, Hitler proclaimed that the 'discovery of the Jewish virus' is one of the 'greatest revolutions the world has seen.' The struggle in which the Nazis were engaged, Hitler said, was similar to the one 'waged by Pasteur and Koch in the last century. How many diseases must owe their origins to the Jewish virus? Only when we have eliminated the Jews will we regain our health.'

2 The bureaucratic efficiency of the Holocaust is often contrasted with the one-on-one killing of the Rwandan genocide. However, this ignores the very efficient use of the radio in the Rwandan case.

3 See my *Difference and Disavowal: The Trauma of Eros* for the fullest explanation of the relation between fetishism and "concreteness," and defense against the *possibility* of meaning. We will return to this topic in the chapter on Weisband (Chapter 4).

4 This was also true in the Rwandan genocide when Hutus who were "Tutsi identified" were also slaughtered.

5 See Chapter 8, "Semelin on Purification and Destruction."

6 On October 28, 2023, three weeks after the Hamas attack in Israel, Benjamin Netanyahu gave a speech in which he referenced the Biblical account of Amalek. It immediately raised an alarm about genocidal intent. Netanyahu's office claimed that he was only referring to Hamas, but it is impossible to read these Biblical passages without seeing the command to destroy not only what was "evil" in Amalek, but *all* the Amalakites.

2 The Holocaust

Zygmunt Bauman's *Modernity and the Holocaust* challenges the assumption that the Holocaust is a "malady" of contemporary civilization. Rather it is civilization's "horrifying, yet legitimate end product" (p. xii). Bauman means "legitimate" in the sense of the lawful unfolding of the very structure of modernity itself. Within what would seem to be the antithesis of a Holocaust is its inevitability. Bauman isolates three characteristics of modernity: the "emancipation" of the modern state, its monopoly on violence, and its "audacious engineering projects" (p. xiii). The "emancipation" of the modern state, i.e., its existence as an entity unto itself, is often, controversially, considered the result of the Peace of Westphalia of 1648, which ended the Thirty Years' War. Whether this is so or not, the principles associated with Westphalia define what Bauman means by "the emancipation of the modern state": the integrity of national borders and noninterference in the internal affairs of the state: in other words, national sovereignty.

National sovereignty is at the heart of the origin of the word "genocide" itself. It was coined by Rafael Lemkin in his 1944 *Axis Rule in Occupied Europe*. His concern with this as yet unnamed phenomenon began in response to (what came to be called) the Armenian genocide, during World War I.

> While studying at the University of Lviv, Raphael Lemkin, a 21-year-old Polish Jew, came across an article on Soghomon Tehlirian. Tehlirian was an Armenian Genocide survivor on trial for the murder of Mehmet Talaat, one of the orchestrators of the Armenian Genocide, who had at the time escaped prosecution. Lemkin asked [his professor] why the Armenians did not have Talaat arrested for the massacre. The professor said there was no law under which he could be arrested. 'Consider the case of a farmer, who owns a flock of chickens,' he said. 'He kills them and this is his business. If you interfere, you are trespassing.' Finding this gap in international law intolerable, Lemkin began work on an international law proposal for this sort of crime.
>
> (Goldsmith, p. 238)[1]

DOI: 10.4324/9781003562870-3

The professor's analogy makes the point that still holds true today: respect of national sovereignty can be license for genocide.

Bauman's "monopoly on violence" is another expression of noninterference in internal affairs. Freud had addressed this issue: "the state has forbidden to the individual the practice of wrongdoing, not because it desires to abolish it, but because it desires to monopolize it" (1915b, p. 279). "Audacious engineering projects" is to be taken metaphorically, for all the technological advances used to dominate nature and to administer the state. The Holocaust, then, uncovers the destructive face of modernity, the "normality" of its functioning. Bauman sees a straight line from Enlightenment Europe's project of rational world domination to the Final Solution; and from the mass production line to the technology of the concentration camp (p. 9). There is no antithesis between civilization and "savage cruelty" (p. 9). Auschwitz "expands the universe of consciousness no less than landing on the moon" (p. 11).

Bauman too considers the normality of perpetrators of genocide:

> That most of the perpetrators of the genocide were normal people, who will freely flow through any known psychiatric sieve, however dense, is morally disturbing. It is also theoretically puzzling, particularly when seen conjointly with the 'normality' of those organizational structures that coordinated actions of such normal individuals.
>
> (p. 19)

Bauman here would need psychoanalytic theory in order to resolve the "puzzle," and to be able to see why it is related to moral disturbance. In the paranoid-schizoid position, the only morality is that of self-defense against an enemy created by projective identification. Once understood in such terms, Bauman's point about organizational structures becomes more compelling. (Recall Kiernan on the pragmatic, rational skills needed to carry out genocide.) Bauman is telling us that the technologically ordered, rational state administration contains within it precisely what the fantasies of the paranoid-schizoid position demand: the skills necessary for genocide. Describing the paranoid-schizoid position, Melanie Klein speaks of the "horrifying" fantasies of the baby trying to destroy the "bad breast" by every means at its disposal (1975, p. 130). For Bauman, modernity itself contains both the impetus and the means to carry this out on a large scale.

Bauman asserts that "...the civilizing process is, among other things, a process of divesting the use and deployment of violence from moral calculus..." (p. 28). Note the irony: what is supposed to be the advance in morality, the "civilizing process," is actually its reverse. In *Civilization and Its Discontents,* once again discussing "the human instinct of aggression and self destruction" (, p. 145), Freud says "Men have gained control over the forces of nature to such an extent that with their help they would have no difficulty in exterminating one another to the last man" (1930, p. 145). The scientific, rational progress of technology becomes a manifestation of the death drive; Freud sees this before the Holocaust, before the atomic bomb; Klein had already articulated universal, primal fantasies of destruction based on the theory of the death drive. This juxtaposition of technological advance, the death drive, and the structure of the paranoid-schizoid position, would be central to Bauman's argument. He might disclaim this, having said that genocide is not a question of "the mysteries of individual psychology," but of social and political mechanisms (p. 33). However, expressions like "mysteries of individual psychology" and "puzzle" (or Marcus' "inconvenient insight' that "accusation in the mirror" expresses an "unconscious impulse") indicate the places where the most crucial questions about genocide do require psychoanalytic explanation.

One of Bauman's essential contributions is his analysis of the status of the Jew in Nazi Germany. He starts from the familiar opposition of "us" and "them" (p. 34). But he goes on to show the internal paradox of this opposition: "The objects of antisemitism occupy as a rule the semantically confusing and psychologically unnerving status of foreigners inside, thereby striding a vital boundary which ought to be clearly drawn and kept intact and impregnable" (p. 34). This is the problem of the opposition of essences that are not to meet, and of the dangerously porous boundary between them. What is foreign should not be inside. If it is inside, it is "psychologically unnerving" because it embodies difference—separation *and* connection, outside *and* inside. This psychic process is then translated into the familiar trope of the Jews with no territory of their own, such that, in Hitler's conception, they must use "indecent, surreptitious and underhanded methods," which made them even more sinister; an enemy never to be pacified, only destroyed (p. 35).

For Bauman, this conception of the Jew began with the separation of Judaism and Christianity. For Christianity the Jews "defied cognitive clarity and the moral harmony of the universe" (p. 37). They were neither heathens nor heretics, but the fathers of Christianity who refused to accept the truth when given the chance, "co-extensive and co-terminal with Christianity" (p. 37). Once Christianity was born of its rejection *by* the Jews, drawing its vitality from this rejection, the Jews were endowed with a "*powerful and sinister fascination*" (p. 38). This picture of the Jew was inherited by modernity. "The concept brought together elements that neither belonged together nor could be reconciled with one another. The sheer incoherence of their conflation" marked them as "fascinating and repulsive" (p. 39). "The conceptual Jew was a semantically overloaded entity, comprising and blending meanings which ought to be kept apart…" (p. 39).

What Bauman calls the "conceptual Jew" is then a version of an idea made material, a fetishistic delusion. But fetishistic delusions are a response to "the reality of difference," which itself irreducibly comprises "meanings which ought to be kept apart"—separation *and* connection. The "incoherence of their conflation" (Bauman) for the anti-Semitic propagandist expresses the unconscious response to this reality, and the compelling need to disavow it by creating apparently orderly oppositions of essences. The "conceptual Jew" demonstrates the necessity of keeping meanings "apart," precisely because their integrity, like identity, is porous. The anti-Semitic propagandist is actually haunted by the unbearable tension that where there is difference, oppositions can meet. The "conceptual Jew" is then the "mind-boggling, uncanny, unreason of deviation…" (p. 39).

"Unreason" is a particularly important word here. It is another way of indicating that genocide is carried out in the name of "reason," i.e., the logic of delusion. But this logic is not simply an aberration of logic as we know it, but like modernity, an extension of it. Logic depends upon the principle of identity: a thing cannot be itself and its opposite. The "conceptual Jew" undermines this logic, is "mind-boggling." It is the possibility of "chaos and devastation" (p. 40). This is why Bauman says that the conceptual Jew is the universal "viscosity" of the Western world (p. 40). In other words, it "oozes," revoltingly, between the terms of what should be pure opposition. The conceptual Jew's "*…very mutli-dimensionality was an extra cognitive incongruence…*" (p. 40). Once opposites have met, what "oozes" can go in any direction, contaminating whatever it encounters. It must be cleaned up if order and reason are to be maintained.

All of this is why Bauman says that in relation to boundary drawing in general, the conceptual Jew cannot be explained in terms of local or coincidental factors (p. 41). "Its incredible capacity of servicing so many different and mutually unrelated concerns and pursuits is rooted precisely in its unique universality, ex-temporality, and ex-territoriality. *It fits so well so many local issues because it is not causally connected with any*" (p. 41). In other words, the "conceptual Jew," as the model for the impossibility of absolutely intact boundaries, is the "uniquely universal" target of genocide, throughout time (ex-temporality) and space (ex-territoriality); at all times and everywhere. Given the universality of genocide then, is something like the "conceptual Jew," the "uniquely universal" model for all targets of genocide?

Bauman uses the word "uncanny" to characterize such "mind boggling" "deviation." Deviation, of course, implies departure from a norm. Before *Group Psychology…*, where Freud spoke of the primally narcissistic violence provoked by racial difference, he had already spoken of the uncanniness of difference, and its link to violence. In *The Taboo of Virginity* (1918), he introduced the famous "narcissism of minor differences":

> primitive man is prey to a perpetual lurking apprehensiveness, just as in the psycho-analytic theory of the neuroses we claim to be the case with people suffering from anxiety neurosis. This apprehensiveness will appear most strongly on all occasions which differ in any way from the usual, which involve something new or unexpected, something not understood or *uncanny*
>
> (p. 196; my emphasis)

This implies a "deviation." The specific possible deviation here is the departure from the norm that a girl remains virgin before marriage, "the taboo of virginity." This seems to be

> so much a matter of course, that we find ourselves almost at a loss if we have to give reasons for this opinion. The demand that a girl shall not bring to her marriage with a particular man any memory of sexual relations with another is, indeed, nothing other than a logical continuation of the right to exclusive possession of a woman
>
> (p. 193)

Note that Freud is speaking of a "right," a legal norm that guarantees "exclusive possession," i.e., nondeviating departure from a fixed place, an unquestionable norm.

What is significant is that Freud goes on to explain the "taboo of virginity" in relation to sexual difference itself.

> Wherever primitive man has set up a taboo he fears some danger and it cannot be disputed that a generalized dread of women is expressed in all these rules of avoidance [taboos of virginity, of menstruation]. Perhaps this dread is based on the fact that woman is different from man, forever incomprehensible and mysterious, strange and therefore apparently hostile.
>
> (p. 197)

If "man" is the norm, then a departure from the norm makes woman not only strange, but hostile, threatening. To use Bauman's terms here, woman exerts a "powerful and sinister fascination." Freud then says:

> it is precisely the minor differences in people who are otherwise alike that form the basis of feelings of strangeness and hostility between them. It would be tempting to pursue this idea and to derive from this 'narcissism of minor differences' the hostility which in every human relation we see fighting successfully against feelings of fellowship and overpowering the commandment that all men should love one another.
>
> (p. 198)

Again using Bauman's terms, Freud here seems to be describing the uncanniness of the "conceptual woman."

Freud later devoted an essay to the uncanny, in German *das Unheimliche*. The essay begins with a discussion of the word itself, which defies the principle of identity because "...among its different shades of meaning the word '*heimlich*' exhibits one which is identical with its opposite, '*unheimlich*'. What is *heimlich* thus comes to be *unheimlich*" (1919, p. 224). Freud then speaks of the experience of the uncanny when one "identifies himself with someone else, so that he is in doubt as to which his self is, or substitutes the extraneous self for his own. In other words, there is a doubling, dividing and interchanging of the self" (p. 234). If the "conceptual victim" of genocide is created by projective identification, by "insertion" of what is both self-destructive and "bad" about oneself into the racial other, then there is an "interchanging" of selves between perpetrator and victim. What is apparently most familiar to me—"myself"—is related to what is most "unfamiliar," and therefore threatening in the other. All the forms of splitting, from physical "setting apart" to destruction, are attempts to disavow this process, which for Bauman reaches its acme in modernity. He says that as modernism triumphed, anti-modernism moved underground as "the acute fear of the void, the never-satiated lust for certainty, paranoic mythologies of conspiracy and the frantic search for ever elusive identity. Anti-modernist phobias were 'unloaded' through channels only modernism could provide" (p. 46).

The "conceptual Jew" then undermines the principle of the modern nation-state's presumed internally consistent identity. Once presumed, the nation-state appears to be "natural": within these borders, we are German, American, etc. However, the very existence of a Jewish diaspora, such that Jews live in, and might become citizens of, many countries, defies the "naturalness of national entities" (p. 55). Nationalists have to "resent the the absorptive powers of their own nations" (p. 55).

Absorptive power, one might say, is the power of "porosity," the internalization of difference, which Freud had called "vital," a manifestation of the life drive—but which will always be met by a dedifferentiating death drive. This is where the "mysteries of individual psychology" meet the behaviors of nations. Just as the "conceptual Woman" is the indispensable condition of a presumed masculinity, and therefore both familiar and unfamiliar, an uncanny threat, so the "conceptual Jew" is the indispensable condition of a presumed national and racial identity, and thus an uncanny threat to the nation itself.

One might wonder: which is the bigger threat? Freud originally spoke of the narcissism of minor differences in relation to sexual difference, which Bauman might say is a matter of "individual psychology." Freud then extended the narcissism of minor differences to both national and racial differences in *Group Psychology.* If the uncanniness of sexual difference is universal in individuals, is the "conceptual Jew" the "conceptual Woman" writ large?[2]

Bauman might disagree. While there have always been forms of segregation of women throughout history, genocide against women *per se* is impossible. If, for man, the uncanny threat of woman as difference cannot be eliminated, is the wish to do so displaced onto the different racial other? Bauman maintains a sharp distinction between racism and "heterophobia," the kind of universal fear of otherness that Freud described in "The Taboo of Virginity." He calls "heterophobia" a "focused" manifestation of the wider phenomenon of the anxiety about having "no control over the situation" (p. 64). He says that "heterophobia" has to be distinguished from "contestant enmity," "the antagonism generated by identity seeking and boundary drawing" (p. 64). But he has also said that the "conceptual Jew" is the possibility of "chaos," the chaos of porous identities and boundaries. What is chaos if not loss of control? The loss of control of uncanniness?

Bauman says more about the controllable. He contends that the German public initially was "unconcerned" about Jews, so that Nazi leaders had to develop policy and ideology (p. 74). This ideology created the "conceptual Jew," who stood between "*...tension ridden reality and the hoped for world of tranquil happiness*" (p. 76). (Recall Kiernan on the idealized, utopian visions of the world to be created by genocide, and the idea of a "purified pleasure ego.") The "conceptual Jew" is then "a product of theory" (p. 79). From the psychoanalytic point of view, "theory" here means fantasy as reality, i.e., delusion. Bauman contends that this is the theory of the Jew as responsible for everything uncontrollable. Hence the familiar trope of the Jews as a supernational elite, the arbiters of hidden power, responsible for "*spontaneous and uncontrollable, but usually unfortunate turns of fate...*" (p. 79). This is the Jew who is to be punished (p. 75), the Jew who is a "virus," another image of the potentially uncontrollable. The specificity of the Holocaust has to take into account that the advances of modernity promise control of the uncontrollable. This is why Bauman argues that to confuse the Holocaust with heterophobia as the "timeless reactions to the strangers ... [in] fairly ubiquitous identity conflicts," is not to see it as rooted in aspects of modern mentality and modern social organizations (p. 81).

I believe that Bauman is both right and wrong here. Right in that the specificity of the Holocaust is its inevitability in the technological advances of modernity in the context of national sovereignty. But wrong in that the Holocaust is indeed rooted in heterophobia, emblematized by Freud as the uncanniness of sexual difference that universally provokes violence.

Another genocide scholar, Anthonie Holslag, has examined the same issues, and come to important conclusions about the role of "woman" in the construction of genocidal ideology. He starts from the now familiar idea that creating an essential identity is the support for the annihilation of whatever seems to "deviate" from that identity (p. 96). Annihilation then supports a new, purified, solidified identity. "Genocide is therefore not only a physical warfare, but also symbolic and mythological warfare. It is war aimed at the destruction of identities for self preservation and self-existence" (p. 96). Holslag cites the work of Gerd Baumann, whose work on genocide emphasizes "identification processes" (p. 97), a psychoanalytic topic if ever there was one. While not referencing psychoanalytic thought, Baumann speaks of "grammars" of identity, and coins the resonant term "baby grammars"—"baby" to indicate a primal, universal process, the kind of processes analyzed by both Freud and Klein. Holslag contends that "baby grammar" is central to genocide:

> Othering, or baby-grammar, is always linked with reverse mirroring [...] Each time we attach a connotation to the Other, we are in essence creating an imaginary Self. If we, for example, perceive the Other as spontaneous, we are implying that we think of ourselves as calculating (negative self-connotation). If we think of the Other as backwards, then we consider ourselves progressive or technologically advanced (positive self-connotation).

> We do not only do this during a crisis, but continuously. It is through this process of mirroring where we draw fictitious lines between groups. According to Baumann all the grammatical structures of identification unravel through the genocidal process.
>
> (p. 98)

Kiernan had already outlined the alternation of fantasies of superiority and inferiority, and introduced "accusation in the mirror" from the Rwandan genocide. "Baby grammar" is another version of it: the "reverse mirroring" in which the "Other," in psychoanalytic terms, embodies what we *are not*, in order to reaffirm what *we are*. Especially, for Klein, to call this "baby grammar" would be entirely accurate; she too is describing a primal sense of "self" through the mirroring process of projective identification. Holslag does briefly reference Italian psychoanalyst Franco Fornari who "states that groups, just like an infant, can get into a 'paranoid-schizoid' position, where the infant or group saves itself by destroying the object by which he feels destroyed" (p. 108).

Holslag does note a disagreement with Gerd Baumann, for whom genocide occurs when identification processes disintegrate. For Holslag it is the opposite: in genocide, one aspect of reverse mirroring becomes more prominent than another in order to "solidify the Self" (p. 97). It seems evident to me that both processes occur simultaneously, as when Zygmunt Bauman speaks of "the frantic search for ever elusive identity." Holslag similarly says:

> During the genocidal process, and during moments of crisis and decivilization, baby-grammar does not disappear, but becomes the central form of grammar where ideas of Self are established. In this sense we are, within the genocidal process, not only essentializing Others, but also creating an essentializing Self.
>
> (pp. 98–99)

The "frantic" search for a "solidified" identity takes its ultimate form in relation to the body itself:

> Power over the body is of special importance here. It is, in the most literal sense, the ultimate power one has over another. This power goes further than bureaucratic and institutional power; it is the power over personhood. In this sense violence is the ultimate method of making baby-grammar physical, tangible, visible. The hegemony of ideas is not just internalized in the minds of perpetrators and even the victimized group, but even more, it becomes (literally) inscribed in the body. It is the ultimate confirmation of the existence of the superior Self. Indeed, it is the physical outcome [...] of reverse mirroring.
>
> (Holslag, pp.103–104)

Bauman, of course, would add to this that modernity itself is the ultimate expression of technological power over the body.

For Holslag, perhaps as opposed to Bauman, the question of power over the body has a crucial link to Woman, and to masculinity as the norm for the solidified self. He refers to all the documentation of "the sexualization of violence," the numerous accounts of public rape, disembowelment of pregnant women, genital mutilation of male corpses, during genocides (p. 107). This is why there is a version of the "conceptual Woman" for Holslag:

> Women thus become the embodied boundaries of the nation-state. Controlling women is controlling the reproduction of identity. This does not explain however the mutilation and the removal of men's genitals [...] I think that in these instances there is another mechanism of identity-destruction at play; it is the literal deprivation of the gender identity of the victimized group and thereby enhancing the masculinity of the aggressors
>
> (p. 107)

The psychoanalytic themes are patent here. For instance, disembowelment of a pregnant woman as the epitome of Klein's idea of getting *inside* the persecutory mother, and destroying her with "every means at one's disposal." Likewise, genital mutilation of dead men as the epitome of Freud's idea that from the male perspective women *embody* uncanniness of difference *and* the "fact of castration." For Holslag, because "genocidal violence is aimed at destroying an identity" (p. 109), there is "a dialectic between micro and macro behaviour, and not a dichotomy," and the "abnormal" can become "normal":

> Genocide is successful when a specific group no longer exists, or even more than that, if not only the nation-state but also the national history is cleansed from this foreign element [...].[3] Through the whole machinery of destruction, we see how a layer of identity of the victimized group is indeed stripped away, to solidify a similar layer into a new image of the Self. Once again, these are *subconscious* actions, partly because the grammars of [Gerd] Baumann are day-to-day processes. They are not 'abnormal' to the perpetrators. The institutionalization of the Other has already taken such a shape, that killing the Other is no longer an abnormal act, but even a communal duty to the dominant culture group. We create our identity without realizing it, over and over again. This is the core of the genocidal process, and also the reason why it is so dangerous and why ordinary men can commit horrendous acts; the processes in which these acts take place, the mechanisms behind the acts, are actually so daily, and grind into society so slowly, that stigmatizing and dehumanizing is normal in our day-to-day behaviour. Baby grammar doesn't become genocidal overnight,

> it is a normal process which first gets formed, slowly turns aggressive, then gets institutionalized and can then be expressed physically.
>
> (pp. 108–109; my emphasis)

Where Holslag says "subconscious" we are saying "unconscious."

Let us return to Bauman, and agreement with his analysis of the Holocaust, while disagreeing with him about genocide in general. He powerfully contends that the Holocaust has made "our Western civilization incomprehensible," because the possibility of the Holocaust is always there (p. 84); "*...the unimaginable ought to be imagined*" (p. 85). But the "unimaginable" of genocide, throughout space and time, has always been there. Bauman knows this: "genocide accompanied human history from the start" (p. 88). But the Holocaust "towers high above past genocidal episodes in the same way as the modern industrial plant towers above the craftman's cottage workshop" (p. 89). But is it an accident that de Las Casas called the extermination of the Indians in Guatemala a "holocaust," as Kiernan noted? The word itself means "burnt offering," and has a long theological history; the OED gives many examples of its use from ancient times onward. ("Shoah" in Hebrew means catastrophe.) Bauman says that the "Holocaust Is a by-product of the modern drive to a fully designed, fully controlled world, once the drive is getting out of control and running wild" (p. 93). When things are "out of control" and "running wild," "baby grammar" is always potentially operative, and put to use in the name of reason and morality themselves. This is why any presumed suppression of the "immanent human propensity to cruelty and violence" (p. 96) is an "illusion" (p. 97). Hence, as "thinking grows more rational, the quantity of destruction increases" (p. 97). Where Bauman says that "Genocide is neither abnormal nor a malfunction of modernity" (p. 114), Holslag says that genocide is the result of identity formation via "baby grammar."

Bauman says that "technical responsibility" (p. 101) is a perversion of responsibility, because it leads to "dehumanization of the objects of bureaucratic operation, which itself is reduced to quantitative measures" (p. 102). Dehumanization has always been central to genocide (vermin, virus, evil, etc.), and it is certainly the case that it became bureaucratized and quantified in the Holocaust. But not only there. Kiernan reports that as the Cambodian genocide turned against the "Vietnamized" Khmers themselves, Pol Pot *calculated* that out of a population of eight million, two million were expendable (Kiernan, p. 553). And even in the Biblical accounts of genocide, before modernity, there are general indications of quantity. When the Old Testament god commands that *all* the Amalekites be killed, so that no memory of them will remain, what is "all," if not an indication of quantity, so that "the national history is cleansed from this foreign element" (Holslag)? Bauman argues that the sovereign power of the modern technical state usurps ethical authority (p. 199), that the nation-state "has no conscience" (p. 86). But does the "sovereign," one true god, of the Old Testament have a conscience when it orders *all* the men, women, and children of the tribes who oppose him to be wiped out? The problem here is the relations of quantification, technology, and sovereignty. Recall Kiernan on Charlemagne, who "had 4,500 Saxon prisoners 'beheaded in a single day,' according to the Royal Frankish Annals. Posing as Israelites in a new promised land, Charlemagne's army had apparently drawn inspiration from the biblical massacres of the Amalekites and Moabites" (p. 64). In his account of the Japanese genocide of the Koreans under the command of Hideyoshi in the 16th century, Kiernan also documents reports of the *number* of Koreans slaughtered (pp. 130–131).[4]

What might be difficult for Bauman is the proximity of his analysis of technological modernity to Heidegger. For Heidegger the essence of technology is the reduction of everything to the quantifiable as "standing reserve":

> As soon as what is unconcealed [*physis*; everything that is] [...] concerns man ... exclusively as standing reserve [...] and man is [...] nothing but the orderer of the standing reserve [...] he comes to the point where he himself will have to be taken as standing reserve. Meanwhile, man, precisely as the one so threatened, exalts himself to the posture of lord to the earth.
>
> (p. 308)[5]

One sees here the logic of simultaneous self-destruction and omnipotence characteristic of Nazism. Bauman here would have ample reason to condemn Heidegger's support of Nazism, and later famous silence about the Holocaust. But Heidegger's understanding of technology does illuminate the Holocaust itself. And one can wonder if Heidegger could have seen the relation between the "immanent human propensity to cruelty and violence" and technology. This integration of quantification and cruelty is contained in Bauman's statement that the cruelest ruler has to defend rationality, the "calculus of costs and effects" (p. 203). The "calculus of costs and effects" also presumes calculability and predictability, humans themselves as quantifiable standing reserve, the obverse of chaos and deviation, the possibility of an omnipotently controlled outcome.

This is where Bauman turns to the question of morality and difference. He sees the moral drive as "autonomous and unpredictable" (p. 214), not subject to the "calculus of costs and effects." It escapes codification, serves no purpose outside itself (p. 214). Hence, if "morality cannot be rationalized, it must be rendered irrelevant or suppressed" (p. 214). In psychoanalytic terms, the inability to rationalize morality is the result of the anxieties of Klein's depressive position, the need to maintain paranoid-schizoid defenses against the realization of the "disaster created by one's own sadism." For Bauman, this is the result of what he calls "adiaphoristic action" (p. 213), i.e., the downplaying of unpredictable, "differentiating, and thus potentially divisive, features." He reminds us that "adiaphoric originally meant a thing declared indifferent by the Church" (p. 215). To him, the

> adiaphorization of human action seems to be a necessary constitutive act of any supra-individual, social totality; [...] society conceived of as an adiaphorizing mechanism offers a much better explanation of the ubiquitous cruelty endemic in human history than does the orthodox theory of the social origin of morality.
>
> (p. 217)

What Bauman calls adiaphorization seems to mean the homogenization, the dedifferentiation, constitutive of a totality. Whatever resists homogenization is "potentially divisive." The mandatory maintenance of homogenization against difference-division justifies cruelty and violence. When Bauman says that this is a better explanation of endemic cruelty throughout history than "the orthodox theory of the social origin of morality," he is implying that a social origin of morality is impossible, if social organizations themselves are adiaphoristic. "The objects of genocide are always a *category*, which obliterates personal differences" (p. 227). Categories themselves are a rational sorting mechanism: this is included, that is not. The *obliteration* of "personal differences" translates the need to annihilate difference itself: difference which is divisive, unpredictable, uncontrollable, and resistant to homogenization. Modern technology makes "adiaphoristic action" "potentially disastrous" (p. 219). Ultimately, this reveals the contradiction within modernity: "The technologically created world can no longer be technologically controlled" (p. 220). But the question remains about how exclusive this is to modernity. Bauman contends that in "pre-modern times" bloody conquests or internecine strife "led on occasion to well-nigh complete self-annihilation of established elites" (p. 111). Would not the "frantic," technological use of genocide to hopelessly attempt to control the uncontrollable, be the "modern" version of "self-annihilation"? Is this not the self and other destructiveness of the death drive in "adiaphoristic action"?

Bauman does open a space for the widest possible thinking about genocide. From a "philosophical"—the quotation marks indicating the thinking of the limits of philosophy—point of view he is raising the question of inevitable recoil from the uncanniness of difference. From the psychoanalytic point of view he is doing the same, whether the question is the threat of "minor differences," or the use of projective identification to create an undifferentiated, mirroring relation between perpetrator and victim. These are not abstract considerations. *Uncountable* people have been murdered because of them.

Notes

1 For an essential account of Lemkin's life and work, see Philippe Sands, *East-West Street*.

2 Donna Maddox, a forensic psychiatrist who testified for the defense in the trial of Dylann Roof gave a detailed account of Roof's somatic delusions. These were mainly associated with his belief that testosterone "pooled" in the left side of his body and

that the right side of his body was "feminine" or a "eunuch." One can consider these delusions in terms of the sexual conflicts of a disturbed adolescent, but they strikingly suggest that Roof's murderous racism was related to an attempt to rid his body of femininity. Roof himself contended that "psychology is a Jewish invention ... and does nothing but invent diseases and tell people they have problems when they don't" (Bass, 2021, p. 291).

3 In the Biblical account, the very existence of the Amalakeites was to be cleansed from memory.

4 In his introduction to *Annihilating Difference*, Hinton cites the *counting* of the victims of slaughter by Genghis Khan's soldiers (p. 7). He says more about counting partly in reference to Bauman: "'Development' requires rational design (and, of course, the centralized control of the modern nation-state); rational design, in turn, requires legible, precise units..." (p. 13). In her study of the Holocaust, *The Spirit in Ashes*, Edith Wyschogrod analogously refers to this logic in relation to Zeno's paradox, the infinite divisibility of integers to which there is no end. Just as there is no end to divisibility, there is no end to countable integers, such that once victims of genocide are *identified*, in a sense given unit status, there is no end to potential, countable victims.

5 Does Heidegger's phrase, man as "lord of the earth," echo the Biblical creation of man in God's image, and then given "dominion" over "all the earth"? (Genesis 1:26). From the psychoanalytic perspective, one would interpret that the men who composed Genesis wished to see themselves as godlike, omnipotent, such that "all the earth" is their standing reserve." Heidegger's point that man himself inevitably becomes a standing reserve certainly suggests the logic of genocide, in which killing large numbers of people is supposed to enhance the dominion of the perpetrators. This is borne out by the precise descriptions of the genocides of the Midianites (Numbers 31) and the Amalekites (1 Samuel 15) commanded by the sovereign, one true God.

3 State Racism

In *Society Must Be Defended,* Michel Foucault provides an analysis of what he calls "state racism." This analysis culminates in a statement about Nazism that is in many ways the complement of Bauman's.

Foucault is a "genealogist" of *power.* Genealogy, for him, is a means to rescue "buried scholarly knowledge and disqualified popular knowledge" from "the tyranny of overall discourses, with their hierarchies" (p. 8). What he calls the "institutionalization of scientific discourses ... embodied in a theoretical-commercial network such as psychoanalysis ... is largely irrelevant" (p. 9). Nonetheless, I hope to show that Foucault's analysis of the role of racism in what he calls "the raw memory of fights" (p. 8) is in fact congruent with psychoanalytic theory.

Foucault asks, "What is power?" He first looks at it in relation to the "classic juridical theory of power" (p. 13). According to him, there

> power is regarded as a right which can be possessed in the way one possesses a commodity, and which therefore can be transferred or alienated [...] through a juridical act [...] Power is the concrete power that any individual can hold, and which he can surrender [...] so as to constitute a power or a political sovereignty [...] political power [...] is modeled on a juridical operation similar to an exchange of contracts.
>
> (p. 13)

This is the view he contests, saying that "there are not many tools for a non-economic analysis of power" (p. 13), and certainly not "the ideas of Hegel, Freud, and Reich that power is that which represses" (p.14). Inverting Clausewitz's famous statement that war is politics by other means, Foucault says that "power is war, the continuation of war by other means" (p. 15). Power is anchored in a relationship of force established in and through war at a historically specifiable moment:

> And while it is true that political power puts an end to war and establishes or attempts to establish the reign of peace in civil society, it certainly does

DOI: 10.4324/9781003562870-4

> not do so in order to suspend the effects of power or to neutralize the disequilibrium revealed by the last battle of the war.
>
> (p. 15)

Power is always operative, and is always a question of war. Historically, there have been different forms of political power/war (p. 16). For Foucault, there was an important permutation of power at the end of the 19th century: "race struggle and class struggle became ... the two great schemata that were used to identify the phenomenon of war and the relationship of force within political power" (p. 19). The relation of "race struggle" to political power is our topic.

Political power is usually conflated with the question of sovereignty. Foucault looks at the understandings of royal power in the Middle Ages, when

> either it had to be demonstrated that royal power was invested in a juridical armature, that the monarch was indeed the living body of sovereignty [...] or it had to demonstrate that the power of the sovereign had to be limited[...] the major or central problem around which the theory of right is organized is the problem of sovereignty
>
> (p. 26)

Foucault will question this centrality of sovereignty to the theory of right. However, we have already seen that it is essential to the understanding of genocide, e.g., in the allegory of the farmer and the chickens as the reason why there was no way to prosecute the Armenian genocide. The farmer has the sovereign right to kill his chickens.

Foucault: "we have to bypass or get around the problem of sovereignty—which is central to the theory of right—and the obedience of individuals who submit to it, and to reveal the problem of domination and subjugation instead of sovereignty and obedience" (p. 27). (The psychoanalyst will immediately wonder whether Foucault is describing the dynamics of sado-masochism: domination and subjugation.) As power, "domination is not a question of one individual over another, one group over another" (p. 29). Rather, power

> circulates. It functions only as part of a chain [...] it is never appropriated in the way wealth or a commodity can be appropriated. Power functions. Power is exercised through networks, and individuals do not simply circulate in these networks; they are in a position to both submit to and exercise this power [...] power passes through individuals. It is not applied to them
>
> (p. 29)

(Again, the psychoanalyst will wonder whether Foucault is describing the dynamics of sado-masochism, in which submission and domination are reversible. We will return to this question in the next chapter.)

Foucault is well known for his work on the disciplinary measures that he says are "the great invention of bourgeois society" (p. 36). He sees the "discourse of discipline" as a "code of normalization that refers to the field of the human sciences and clinical knowledge" (p. 38). We have already encountered Bauman on deviation and norm. Foucault proposes that "… we should be looking for a new right that is both anti disciplinary and emancipated from the principle of sovereignty" (p. 40). Genocide, one might say following Foucault, is the ultimate disciplining of deviation justified by "the human sciences and clinical knowledge," and made legal by the principle of unlimited sovereignty.

Asking himself whether war is the "matrix for analyzing techniques of domination" (p. 46), Foucault says that "law is born of real battles, burning towns, ravaged fields, the innocent dead" (p. 50). He is telling us that law and sovereignty *exist* because of real battles, burning towns, ravaged fields and the innocent dead. The theory of sovereignty attempts to show how "a power can be constituted, not exactly in accordance with the law," but in accordance with a "certain basic legitimacy that is more basic than any law and that allows laws to function as such" (p. 44), a legitimacy inextricably founded on violence. Freud gives a "mythical" account of the same process in *Totem and Taboo,* where the murder of the primal father by his sons is the origin of law, i.e., the necessity of the rule that the sons may not in turn kill each other. And we have already seen (in our last chapter) that Freud says laws against violence permit the state to monopolize it. Further back, the Biblical commandment against killing reserved a right to genocide for the unlimited sovereignty of the one, true god.

When Foucault says that war "only ends with "our victory" over "the enemies who face us [and] still pose a threat to us" (p. 51), he is saying that there will always be a threatening enemy. Why would this not be related to the way the death drive is inevitably projected onto or into an other for both Freud and Klein, and therefore to the irreducibility of racial hatred and violence? In a passionate paragraph, Foucault concludes that there is a:

> fundamental and permanent irrationality, a crude and naked irrationality, but which proclaims the truth; and, higher up, we have a fragile rationality, a transitory rationality, which is always compromised and bound up with illusion and wickedness. Reason is on the side of wild dreams, cunning and the wicked. At the opposite end of the axis, you have an elementary brutality: a collection of deeds, acts, and passions, and cynical rage … Truth is therefore on the side of unreason and brutality; reason, on the other hand, is on the side of wild dreams and wickedness
>
> (p. 55)

Foucault here outlines many of the same themes we have taken from psychoanalysis. He begins with "fundamental and permanent irrationality." In our terms, these are the basic, "fundamental" unconscious processes, the permanent irrationality of primary process, wish fulfillment as tension reduction. This irrationality "proclaims the truth." This is the mechanism Freud describes for psychosis, the necessity to find proof in the world of the veracity, the truthfulness, of delusion—primary process in the waking state. When Foucault speaks of "wild dreams," he clearly intends waking, violent fantasies of destruction. However, one can take this in Freud's sense as the use of primary process in waking life to create delusions. As Foucault says, this results in a "compromised" rationality, the apparent logic of illusion (delusion). And it is "bound up with wickedness"; primal violence against difference, the mandatory attack on the persecutory object of the paranoid-schizoid position, an elementary, enraged "brutality." Truth, again, is "unreason," or the "reason" of delusion. Reason itself then operates to actualize "wild dreams and wickedness," using secondary process, practical, technical, rationality in order to execute "war" in Foucault's general sense.

How does this produce the theory of "state racism"?

Foucault contends that from the 17th century, war is translated into the specific form of a race that divides society in a binary mode (pp. 59–60). It must be recalled that "race" then meant the binary opposite of whoever one was at war with, the enemy, and not necessarily the ethnic difference with which we associate it today. For the English, the Irish were a different race. However, when the conception of power changed in the 19th century into control of populations, power became "*bio*-power," power over life itself. This produced the "absolutely new discourse" of *bio*logical-social racism (p. 61), which produced a new conception of race:

> the other race is basically not the race that came from elsewhere or that was, for a time, triumphant and dominant, but that it is a race that is permanently, ceaselessly infiltrating the social body, or which is, rather, constantly being re- created in and by the social fabric. In other words, what we see as a polarity, as a binary rift within society, is not a clash between two distinct races. It is the splitting of a single race into a superrace and a subrace. To put it a different way, it is the reappearance, within a single race, of the past of that race. In a word, the obverse and the underside of the race reappears within it.
>
> (p. 61)

Again, we find a description of the "logic" of racism very close to what we have elaborated thus far. First, the discourse of contamination, infiltration of the "social body," i.e., fantasies of the nation as a body, permanently at risk of disease. But what is the disease? One might call it an autoimmune disorder, a disease ceaselessly created by the body itself. Hence, what appears to be a binary "rift" within the "body politic" is actually that body's "splitting" of itself into a superior and inferior race, the "reappearance" of the *past* of that race. From the psychoanalytic point of view, this is the *past* of the creation of the purified pleasure ego, which expels its own tensions onto an external object which it then "hates, abhors, and attempts to destroy," even at the risk of its own self preservation. Analogously, it is the creation of a persecutory object which is a permanent threat. The "obverse and underside of the race appears within it."

This process, in turn, is conceived in terms of norm and deviation:

> The discourse of race struggle—which when it first appeared and began to function in the seventeenth century, was essentially an instrument used in the struggles waged by decentered camps—will be reentered and will become the discourse of power itself. It will become the discourse of a centered, centralized, and centralizing power. It will become the discourse of a battle that has to be waged not between races, but by a race that is portrayed as the one true race, the race that holds power and is entitled to define the norm, and against those who deviate from the norm, against those who pose a threat to the biological heritage. At this point, we have all those biological racist discourses of degeneracy, but also all those institutions within the social body which make the discourse of race struggle function as a principle of exclusion and segregation, and ultimately, as a way of normalizing society
>
> (p. 61)

"Decentered camps": for example, the English and Irish, two apparently distinct bodies at war. But once it is a question of life itself, the more control over life is "centralized," the more it becomes a question of a racial norm. A central power defends its normativity against the contaminating "subrace" it has created from within itself, the "degenerate" race that must be kept apart.

This, then, creates "state racism":

> We have to defend society against all the biological threats posed by the other race, the subrace, the counterrace that we are, despite ourselves bringing into existence. At this point, the racist thematic is no longer a moment in the struggle between one social group and another; it will promote the global strategy of social conservativisms. At this point [...] we see the appearance of a State racism: a racism that society will direct against itself, against its own elements and its own products. This is the internal racism of permanent purification, and it will become one of the basic dimensions of social normalization.
>
> (pp. 61–62)

The "internal racism of permanent purification" is the response that Bauman has already analyzed as the reaction to the "foreigner within." Foucault says the same, speaking of "the idea that foreigners have infiltrated this society, the theme of the deviants who are this society's by-products" (p. 81). This is the autoimmune response to "society" itself, the creation of "the subrace the counterrace that we are, despite ourselves bringing into existence." For

Bauman this was the "conceptual Jew." In Cambodia, there were "Vietnamized" Khmers, and in Rwanda "Tutsified" Hutus. According to Kiernan:

> In Rwanda, majority Hutu moderate politicians were only the first to be killed. The short-lived Hutu Power regime then quickly killed thousands more Hutu, especially intellectuals [...] accusing them of lacking zeal for its larger campaign to exterminate the Tutsi [...], all of which had to be 'cleansed'.
>
> (Kiernan, p. 559)

Foucault puts it this way:

> the State is, and must be, the protector of the integrity, the superiority, and the purity of the race [...] the discourse of race [...] [is used] [...] to preserve the sovereignty of the State, a sovereignty [...] guaranteed [...] by medico-normalizing techniques [...] State sovereignty thus becomes the imperative to protect the race.
>
> (p. 82)

Nazism takes up the State racism responsible for the biological protection of the race, and combines it with the prophetic discourse of race struggle, the struggle of a Germanic race enslaved by the Slavs, the treaty of Versailles, etc. (p. 82). Its discourse of "races in struggle ... [is] definitively detached ... from a historico-juridical consciousness centered on sovereignty" (p. 83). Foucault here is justifying his argument against the question of unlimited or limited sovereignty, the "juridical" question of sovereignty, and extending the logic of bio-power, exemplified by the discourse of "race struggle," or really war. This will be the discourse of the existence of a "master race" (Aryan, Hutu, Khmer, etc.), but a race always threatened by a contaminating "other" (Jew, Tutsi, Vietnamese), over which one must gain control. Even if not sovereignty in the classical juridical sense, it is still a form of sovereignty, what Foucault will call "the sovereign right to kill" (p. 260). From the psychoanalytic point of view, the question of sovereignty would be irreducible, because it is a manifestation of the "frantic" effort to gain omnipotent control over the uncontrollable infecting subrace created by the State itself.

Addressing the question of millennial anti-Semitism, Foucault contends that until the emergence of bio-power in the 19th century, what he calls "traditional anti-Semitism" had little relation to the idea of the State itself as a war between binary groups.

> The old religious type of anti-Semitism was reutilized by State racism only in the nineteenth century, or at the point when the State had to look like, function and present itself as the guarantor of the integrity and purity of the race, and had to defend it against the race or races that were infiltrating it, introducing harmful elements into its body, and which therefore had to be

> driven out for both political and biological reasons [...] At this point the Jews came to be seen as [...] a race that was present within all races, and whose biologically dangerous character necessitated a certain number of mechanisms of rejection and exclusion on the part of the State.
>
> (p. 89)

The Jew as a biologically dangerous race "present in all races" is, again, Bauman's "conceptual Jew," which I believe to be at the heart of genocidal delusion (the "conceptual Tutsi," the "conceptual Vietnamese," etc.).

Bio-power, state racism, for Foucault, is the transformation of sovereignty into the power over life and death. "Sovereign power's effect on life is exercised only when the sovereign can kill. The very essence of the right of life and death is actually the right to kill" (p. 240). Which is why bio-power is "always tipped in favor of death" (p. 239). To protect the superior race, it must be "purified"; the dangerous subrace must be killed. "The very essence of the right of life and death is actually the right to kill" (p. 240). And in the 19th century this was supported by all the medical, clinical discourses about race and contamination itself (Hitler's references to Koch and Pasteur, both of the 19th century):

> beneath the dramatic and somber absolute power that was the power of sovereignty, and which consisted in the power to take life, we now have the emergence, with this technology of bio-power, of this technology of power over the population as such [...] [Biopower] is continuous, scientific, and it is the power to make live.
>
> (p. 247)

I think that what Foucault is calling bio-power is a "permutation" of the entire delusional logic of purification as elimination. The Old Testament god commands the elimination of the Amalekites in order to erase "evil." Where Bauman analyzes the Holocaust in relation to technological modernity, Foucault proposes state racism. Both can be understood to illustrate the way in which political transformation and technological advance can be used to buttress the mechanisms of the paranoid-schizoid position, the "final solution" to the existence of the persecutory object.

If traditional sovereignty is waning, and disciplinary or regulatory power increasing, Foucault asks, "how will the power to kill and the function of murder operate in this technology of power?" (p. 254). "Given that this power's objective is essentially to make live, how can it let die? ... It is at this point, I think, that racism intervenes" (p. 254). Racism itself was not new; what was new was the use to which it was put:

> the emergence of this bio-power [...] inscribes [racism] in the mechanisms of the State [...] the modern State can scarcely function without becoming involved with racism at some point [...] What in fact is racism? It is primarily

> a way of introducing a break into the domain of life that is under power's control: the break between what must live and what must die.
>
> (p. 254)

Foucault has already described the self-division of one "race" into superior and inferior "races." The sovereign right to kill expands: the more you kill, the more deaths you will cause, the more you will live. This is war: in order to live you must kill your enemies. But this is a "completely new" form of war in that it is biological. "The death of the bad race, the inferior race, the degenerate race, makes life healthier and purer" (p. 255). The presumption is that protection of the life of the superior, threatened, race promises a kind of utopian (Kiernan) longevity. The "thousand-year Reich" will be "*Judenrein*," purified of Jews.

> In a normalizing society, race or racism is the precondition that makes killing possible ... racism is the indispensable precondition that allows someone to be killed ... Once the State functions in the bio-power mode, racism alone can justify the murderous function of the State.
>
> (p. 256)

Here, Foucault is emphatic: "Racism [in its relation to the State] first develops with colonization, or in other words with colonizing genocide" (p. 257). While there is no doubt that colonization produced massive genocides, genocide itself did not await Foucault's State racism. Perhaps what he calls "State racism" is a version of genocidal "logic" itself. Bauman understood this logic as "adiaphoristic action," the downplaying of unpredictable, "differentiating, and thus potentially divisive, features," which he said was "a necessary constitutive act of any supra-individual, social totality," an "explanation of the ubiquitous cruelty endemic in human history" (p. 213). If differentiation itself is constitutive of identity, but also inevitably provokes an autoimmune response to the division of identity, State racism is another form of "adiaphoristic action." Destruction of difference as self-destruction—the death-drive.

Foucault too, develops an argument about genocide and self-destruction: "the most murderous States are also, of necessity, the most racist." The

> destruction of other races was therefore not really the destruction of other races. The destruction of other races was one aspect of the project, the other being to expose its own race to the absolute and universal threat of death.
>
> (pp. 258–259)

Why? Because "exposing the entire population to universal death was the only way it could truly constitute itself as a superior race and bring about its definitive regeneration once other races had been either exterminated or enslaved forever" (p. 260). This brings Foucault to the logical conclusion of his entire analysis: "Nazi society ... has generalized bio-power in an absolute sense, but ... has also generalized the sovereign right to kill ... *We have an absolutely racist State, an absolutely murderous State, and an absolutely suicidal state*" (p. 260; my emphasis). Kiernan made a similar point: "In the case of the Hutu of Rwanda, as with the Khmer majority under DK [Democratic Kampuchea] and even the Germans under Nazism, the subjection of individuals to the overwhelming interest of their 'race' only made them more vulnerable to violence purportedly 'protecting' them from racial contamination" (p. 559). Foucault: "Nazism alone took the play between the sovereign right to kill and the mechanisms of bio power to this paroxysmal point. But this play is in fact inscribed in the workings of all States" (p. 260). Foucault asks himself: "How can one both make a bio power function and exercise the rights of war, the rights of murder and the function of death, without becoming racist? That was the problem and that, I think, is still the problem" (p. 263).

Will it always be the problem? To the extent that Foucault's analysis of sovereignty and racism corresponds to the dynamics of the purified pleasure ego, the paranoid-schizoid position, and the death drive, the answer is inevitably "yes." If so, then any prevention of genocide must take such sobering truth into account. If it does not, then all the cries of "never again," will constantly have to face that they are delusion, a belief that replaces an intolerable reality, a delusion that prevents understanding of the equally delusional structure of "state racism" and genocide itself.

4 The "Macabresque"

Edward Weisband's *The Macabresque. Human Violation and Hate in Genocide, Mass Atrocity, and Enemy-Making* extends Foucault's analysis of Nazism, but in a way Foucault probably would contest, because of his reliance on psychoanalytic thought. Weisband writes: "Freudian and post-Freudian discourses have become so discredited … among the empirical social sciences … that studies of genocide and mass atrocity falter on the failures of *interdisciplinarity* over apparent fears of *multidisciplinarity*" (p. 98; author's emphasis). Echoing some of the themes we have already encountered:

> Objectification, along with dehumanization, demonization, and essentialization, thus represents the way of depicting relationships devoid of benevolence, sympathy, empathy, or even pity […] Related to this issue is the question of narcissism and of 'minor differences' long familiar to students of Freudian psychoanalysis. Some of the most horrendous outbreaks of genocidal outrage appear to emerge in political cultures assailed by 'minor' identitarian differences
>
> (p. 52)

The juxtaposition of essentializing relations devoid of pity with the narcissism of minor differences integrates basic ideas of Freud and Klein. Freud postulated a primally aggressive response to sexual and racial difference. Klein theorized this aggression in terms of the mechanisms of the paranoid-schizoid position (projection of the death drive, splitting, projective identification), in which the "disaster created by one's own sadism" does not exist; hence, no sympathy, empathy, or pity. Weisband's topic too, is sadism, which he calls the "macabresque." He is taking an in-depth look at the cruel, sadistic, and *pleasurable* aspects of genocide.

Weisband defines the macabresque as the "performative transgressions and *aesthetics* of human violation in genocide and mass atrocity" (p. 7; my emphasis). He knows that it is "commonplace to assert that mostly ordinary citizens are the main practitioners of genocide and mass atrocity" (p. 7). But what he calls "aesthetics" implies sensation (in the etymological sense)

DOI: 10.4324/9781003562870-5

and appreciation, art, and pleasure (in the everyday sense). He asks us not to take the apparent normality of those who commit genocide at face value, concentrating on what they evidently *desire,* even if that desire is unacknowledged—a basically psychoanalytic way of proceeding. There is a confirmation of Weisband's emphasis on normality masking sadistic desire in Arendt's *Eichmann in Jerusalem*. She writes that in preparation for the trial, "Half a dozen psychiatrists certified him as 'normal' ... a man with very positive ideas" (p. 25). But after the trial:

> revelations in the *Saturday Evening Post* of things he [Gideon Hausner, the main prosecutor] 'could not bring out at the trial' have contradicted the information given informally in Jerusalem. Eichmann, we are now told, had been alleged by the psychiatrists to be 'a man obsessed with a dangerous and insatiable urge to kill,' a 'perverted sadistic personality'
>
> (p. 26)

From the outset, starting with Diamond, we have seen the amalgam of "instinct" and "ethics" in genocide. Weisband too, sees an "analytical link between willful or disordered perpetrator desire" and "moralism, self-sacrifice, and a perverted sense of heroism" (p. 9). One might say that he is looking at the global moralism of Himmler on the obligation to "destroy this people who want to destroy us," or the individual "heroism" of Dylann Roof's attempt to start a race war, and is then asking about their implicit sadism. The question for Weisband is why such sadism always *accompanies* genocide:

> Cruelty in the macabresque theaters of performative transgression is always a *surplus,* always beyond strategic necessity, because it originates in the perpetrators' unconscious and disordered desires [...] Noir ecstasy in the macabresque seeks its own set of enjoyments that conceal the sources of desiring from those who are the desiring subjects, the perpetrators themselves
>
> (p. 14; author's emphasis)
>
> This "surplus enjoyment" of "concealed" "noir ecstasy" allows
>
> perpetrators to revel in their absolute power, but simultaneously, to project hatred, revenge, and revulsion onto their victims, who are reified and thus made to appear, at first in fantasy but eventually in ideological constructions, as the very incarnation of the shame, humiliation, and loss against which the perpetrators also seek to defend
>
> (p. 10)

Such projected intolerable knowledge is a version of "accusation in the mirror." Weisband's term is "mimetic rivalry" (p. 25). The "rival" embodies what the perpetrator cannot tolerate about himself. We have already alluded to Freud's idea of a purified pleasure ego that projects the "bad" that it cannot tolerate in itself onto an external, and then hated, object, which it seeks to destroy. Weisband expands that idea. Projection of intolerable shame, humiliation, and loss, also creates a rival that is a version of oneself, hence a *mimetic* rival. To subdue or eliminate the mimetic rival then permits the perpetrator to "revel" in "absolute power"—omnipotence for psychoanalysis. Foucault would not use a psychoanalytic term like "omnipotence"; however, like Weisband, he did use "absolute": Nazi Germany was "absolutely racist, absolutely murderous, and absolutely suicidal." Weisband will come back to precisely this, the pleasure in, and autoimmunity of, omnipotence, fantasized absolute power.

> What perpetrators apparently seek [...] [is] to share in shared desire with those of the same blood, race, and cultural or political identity, not for ideological reasons as such, but as an unconscious means of attaining transcendence beyond finitude and mortality.
>
> (p. 25)

What is apparently ideological is the enactment of shared omnipotent fantasy, "transcendence beyond finitude and mortality." (Recall Kiernan on the utopian visions of genocide.) The support of shared omnipotent fantasy is the "mimetic rival" as the *necessary* threat to the desire for "blood and belonging" (p. 26). Necessary because elimination of the rival seems to guarantee transcendence, blood, and belonging. But, the desire for "blood and belonging" is itself a "substitute," a substitute for what Lacan calls *jouissance*, which is

> a psychic force that is tantalizing, even titillating, but also shocking and repulsive given its power to destroy the sense of individuation, even personality. The more one has of *jouissance*, the closer one comes to it, the less one can bear or support it ... This produces a primordial yearning in surrogacy for what Lacan calls *objet a*, that is, objects of desire alternative to *jouissance*, comprising psychic modes of desire and desiring, not merely in terms of acquisition, but, rather, in terms of subjectivation and human development.
>
> (p. 26)

Weisband cites Bruce Fink, noted translator of Lacan, on *objet a*: it allows the split subject of the unconscious to sustain the illusion of wholeness, to ignore division (p. 26). *Objet a* as the desire for intact "blood and belonging," creates an identity constituted by the delusion that the division, the difference, that constitutes identity has been expelled, which is why the mimetic rival is necessary. Weisband has already referred to (Freud's) "minor identitarian differences." Bauman had spoken of "adiaphoristic action" (p. 213), the fantasized control of unpredictable, "differentiating, and thus potentially divisive, features." Weisband states that under conditions of "mimetic rivalry and extreme anxiety over threatened social loss or political dissolution" (p. 27), the narcissism of minor differences leads "desire to enter darker diabolical realms, where *objet a* travels psychically ever nearer emotionally to the forbidden territories of lost ecstasy and proscribed enchantment" (p. 27).

It is this progression toward *jouissance* that explains the "chameleon-like" behavior of perpetrators, their ordinariness before and after genocide (p. 30), as in the case of Eichmann. Weisband cites Stephen Frosh: "What, if there is no element of fantasy involved, can explain the frenzy, *the willingness to demolish the self as the other*?' (cited, p. 31; my emphasis). This "frenzy," Lacan's *jouissance*, is the siren call of self-other destruction—the origin of aggression in the death drive.

Weisband has emphasized sadism, but his understanding of "self-other destruction" also implies masochism. In *Beyond the Pleasure Principle*, Freud had mentioned the possibility of a primacy of masochism in relation to the death drive, reversing his previous conception of the primacy of sadism. He returned to the relation of the death drive to masochism in *The Economic Problem of Masochism* (1924c). In that paper he defines "primary masochism" as the portion of the death drive that remains within every individual, and is fused with libido (1924, pp. 163–164). Freud's primary masochism is very close to Lacan's *jouissance*. If one integrates this idea with Weisband on mimetic rivalry, then the more the death drive is projected, the more than one approaches *jouissance*, the greater the intensity of primary masochism, the arousal of the death drive fused with libido. Hence, the sadism and cruelty of the "macabresque" and the masochistic erotics of self-destruction.

In *The Economic Problem of Masochism*, Freud had also spoken of "moral masochism," the drive to abnegation in the name of ethics. This becomes another shared desire of the perpetrators. Weisband says that such a group is

> sealed in the blood bonds of honor that transform absolute power as an end itself into the badge of duty [...] that is into a realm of self-deception in which the vilest forms of cruelty loom as the heights of supererogatory heroism.
>
> (p. 99)

The amalgam of instinct and ethics, or of *objet a* and heroism, produces a libidinal autoimmune response, the ecstasy of destruction of self as other. Weisband cites Elizabeth Young-Bruehl:

> Projection theory [...] helps to explain the virulence of genocide and mass atrocity. In this analytical perspective, hatred represents the consequence of resisting guilt [i.e., Klein's idea that the anxieties of the depressive position lead to paranoid-schizoid regression]: the more the guilt, the deeper the projected hatred and reification. As in the case of some forms of cancer, cells that kill originate in the immune system
>
> (cited, p. 106)[1]

Mimetic *rivalry* creates the victim. Within the perpetrator group there is also mimetic *desire*: one desires what the many desire, one desires the desirable (p. 109), the desire for "blood and belonging"—*objet a*. In fantasy, the mimetic rival, the threat to blood and belonging, must not only be punished but also *"seen to be punished"* (p. 111; author's emphasis). This is the aesthetics of genocide, the theater of violation, the struggle over domination and submission, whose ultimate aim is to exert *power* (my emphasis, to recall Foucault) over the rival. The visibility of violation forces the victim to betray himself: "It is as if in their self-betrayal victims are able to bestow the magic or mystery of their *jouissance* into the life-blood of perpetrators who live in the social fantasies of willed self-deception" (p. 111). "A critical dimension of the macabresque is its exhibitionism, the fact that when genocide and mass atrocity unfold, the perpetrators set the stage for each other to witness their sadistic practices of humiliating their victims and making them suffer torture, torment, and agony" (p. 29). As in the reversal of sadism and masochism, there is reversal of voyeurism and exhibitionism in the macabresque, underscoring "the voyeuristic and exhibitionistic behaviors of perpetrators. When they act they wish to be seen, by other perpetrators, by the victims themselves, and in some cases by bystanders" (p. 32)

Without realizing it, in his discussions of reversible sadism and masochism, exhibitionism and voyeurism, Weisband has taken the macabresque into the heart of difficult, but essential, aspects of Freud's theory. In addition to the theory of the purified pleasure ego, in *Instincts and Their Vicissitudes*, Freud took up the themes of sadism and masochism, and exhibitionism and voyeurism, as manifestations of "polymorpously perverse" infantile sexuality. Infantile sexuality by definition comprises drives that occur as pairs of opposites: one side active and the other passive. But these opposites are not *essential* opposites, because the active can always become the passive and vice versa. This is why Freud hypothesizes the existence of "primary, intermediate" phases of the drives, the common root of what can become *reversibly* active and passive. In such primary intermediate phases, active and passive themselves are indistinguishable, because the drive is acting upon itself. It is auto-affective. Holslag, we have seen, elaborated Gerd Baumann's concept of "baby grammar," in which identity is the result of "reverse mirroring." (If I am good, you are bad.) Weisband's use of sadism-masochism and exhibitionism-voyeurism then puts infantile sexuality into "baby grammar," the macabresque pleasure of auto-affective creation of identity via mirroring.

The death drive itself is auto-affective, *self*-destructive. Hence, the comparison to autoimmunity. The mimetic rival is the persecutory object created by the projection of one's own self-destructiveness. When the narcissism of minor differences provokes inevitable, primal violence, and when perpetrators collectively desire something that approaches *jouissance*, sadism and masochism, exhibitionism and voyeurism, join perpetrator and victim into a frenzy of self and other destructiveness. Again, Foucault on Nazism: absolutely racist, absolutely murderous, absolutely suicidal. Weisband: "Foucault brings us closer to an understanding of how normalizing bio-power becomes not only racist but profoundly suicidal once it becomes genocidal and engages in mass atrocity ... power becomes its own worst enemy and nightmare" (p. 42). However, within that nightmare, one finds the apotheosis of auto-affective, unspeakable desire. This is Weisband's expansion of Foucault.

All of which must be integrated with the question of normality. Weisband asks crucial questions:

> If perpetrators acting in groups demonstrate 'normality,' what is in the nature of normalcy that permits those who perpetrate the macabresque to be considered 'normal'? And if what perpetrators do is to be considered part of normal human personality, how do perpetrators envision or represent themselves to themselves—in their normality?
>
> (p. 135)

Answers to these questions are complex. We will take them one at a time.

The first question concerns normality and groups. Weisband cites Kleinian analyst Hanna Segal:

> 'Our psychotic parts are merged into our group identity, and we do not feel mad since our views are sanctioned by the group.' [...] Segal underscores the phenomenon of 'splitting' to emphasize the parallel functioning of psychotic and non-psychotic behavior within large groups
>
> (p. 157)

As a Kleinian, Segal understands the defenses of the paranoid-schizoid position as the psychotic possibilities present in everyone. She makes the simple point that group sanction of the madness of genocide would allow group members to feel "normal": if everyone does it, it must be right. But there is more to the simultaneous functioning of psychotic and nonpsychotic mechanisms.

Wilfred Bion, another eminent Kleinian, made a fundamental contribution to this question in an early paper, which Segal knew. He is dealing with an aspect of the paranoid-schizoid position first discussed by Klein. In her paper on projective identification Klein said that the dominance of that defense produces not only distortion of reality, as one always finds in psychosis, but also "an omnipotent denial of psychic reality" (1986, p. 182). In other words, there is no question of an inner life, of fantasies, anxieties, defenses, etc. Bion took this further. Extending Klein on projective identification, splitting, and the attack on one's own mind, Bion speaks of "a minute splitting of ... that part of the personality that is concerned with awareness of internal and external reality, and the expulsion of these fragments so that they enter into or engulf their objects" (p. 266). For example, in Himmler's conviction that it was morally necessary to protect the German people against the Jews who wanted to destroy them, following Bion, one can say that Himmler's self-confident rationality is actually an attack on his own mind. He had to know that Jews constituted a tiny proportion of the German population, and could not possibly destroy it. But there is clearly a mad, omnipotent wish to destroy in his own mind—but not from his point of view. Instead, this wish engulfs his "objects": the Jews are madly destructive. Thus, Bion speaks of "a preponderance of destructive impulses" and a "dread of imminent annihilation" (p. 266), all of which are evident in Himmler's speech—but not for him.

Elaborating on the simultaneous functioning of psychotic and nonpsychotic parts of the personality, Bion turns to Freud. Freud developed his own theory of splitting late in his life. It is not the same as Klein's. Rather it concerns Bion's topic here, splitting of the ego such that it simultaneously knows and does not know an aspect of reality. Bion cites Freud's final thought about psychosis; even in extreme cases, there is always a splitting of the ego, so that one part of its remains in contact with reality. He integrates this with his understanding of projective identification:

> On this fact, that the ego retains contact with reality, depends the existence of a non psychotic personality parallel with, but obscured by, the psychotic personality [...] the withdrawal from reality is an illusion, not a fact, and arises from the deployment of projective identification against the mental apparatus
>
> (p. 267)

Bion here is dealing with the clinical problem of treatment of the psychotic patient, in which the nonpsychotic part of the personality is projected into the analyst. The analyst is to contain reality, while the patient can withdraw from it. In the genocidal situation, I believe it is the reverse. As in Himmler's speech, it is the madly destructive part of the personality that is projected into the object—the Jews want to destroy us—so that the rest of the personality is "normal," apparently nonpsychotic. As we saw with Bauman, this is what potentiates the use of rational skill to carry out the mad genocidal project.

Weisband' second question is about how perpetrators represent themselves to themselves as normal. "Studies of Nazi elite and rank and file confirm the normality thesis: they were not psychotic or severely disturbed or overwhelmed by sadism or aggression. Rather they showed rigid, eccentric, prejudiced thinking" (p. 136). We have just seen that the apparent normality is the result of projective identification of the psychotic part of the personality. But given what Weisband has said about the approach to *jouissance*, about sadism and masochism, one can wonder how to reconcile such desires with normal, but "rigid, eccentric, prejudiced thinking." Weisband's answer begins with the work of Peter Fonagy on "failure of mentalization." By this, Fonagy means something like what Klein meant by the attack on psychic reality, the conviction that one has no internal states. For Fonagy this is not the result of paranoid-schizoid mechanisms, but of a disturbed relation between baby and mother. The baby does not find itself in the mother's mind, but rather finds the mother herself (cited, p. 138). The mother does not convey understanding of the baby, but only of herself. Such a baby then does not develop a sense of its own internal life; there is a "failure of mentalization." The result is that the "internal and external become mutually implicated" (p. 135).

We have already seen other accounts of such a process. The purified pleasure ego creates a relation to the external that is a projection of its own internal states. Projective identification and Holslag's baby grammar do the same. Returning to Hanna Segal, Weisband cites her on "symbolic equation" (p. 165), the dedifferentiation of symbol and symbolized as a result of projective identification. For Segal, group beliefs are "then *concretized* by means of political and social ideologies, or reified forms of language that narcissistically endow human physicality—that is, bodily, skin or corporeal difference in general—with hatred, often in ways parallel to discursive or ideologically constituted forms of political self-adoration" (p. 166; my emphasis). While there would be disagreement between Fonagy and these more psychodynamic accounts, all are describing the pattern of rigid, eccentric conflation of internal and external as if there is no such conflation. It becomes concretely *true* that the Jews want to destroy us, that Tutsis are vermin, that Vietnamization contaminates Khmer identity. What is concretely true is normal. To indulge in macabresque pleasure then is not cruel, not sadistic, not exhibitionistic—while of course it is. The "disordered desires" of perpetrators can be both gratified and denied. As Weisband has said: "Noir ecstasy in the macabresque seeks its own set of enjoyments that conceal the sources of desiring from those who are the desiring subjects, the perpetrators themselves" (p. 14).

Freud describes an analogous process in his posthumous "Splitting of the Ego in the Process of Defense." He is speaking of typical early conflicts between desire and prohibition:

> Let us suppose, then, that a child's ego is under the sway of a powerful instinctual demand which it is accustomed to satisfy and that it is suddenly frightened by an experience which teaches it that the continuance of this satisfaction will result in an almost intolerable real danger. It must now decide either to recognize the real danger, give way to it and renounce the instinctual satisfaction, or to disavow reality and make itself believe that there is no reason for fear, so that it may be able to retain the satisfaction [...] But in fact the child takes neither course, or rather he takes both simultaneously, which comes to the same thing. He replies to the conflict with two contrary reactions, both of which are valid and effective. On the one hand, with the help of certain mechanisms he rejects reality and refuses to accept any prohibition; on the other hand, in the same breath he recognizes the danger of reality, takes over the fear of that danger as a pathological symptom and tries subsequently to divest himself of the fear [...] Both of the parties to the dispute obtain their share [...] But everything

> has to be paid for in one way or another, and this success is achieved at the price of a rift in the ego which never heals but which increases as time goes on
>
> (1940, pp. 275–276)

What "conceals" the perpetrators' desires from themselves is the concretization of thought as a result of the kind of process Freud describes here. The perpetrator unconsciously seeks gratification of macabresque desire, while simultaneously believing that he does not, that he is only acting sensibly. Macabresque desire makes sense, is normal. One is not being cruel, one is doing the necessary, even the ethical. "Perpetrators ... envision themselves as acting in the name of personal self-sacrifice while psychically gripped by perverse sadism" (p. 172). The self-sacrifice demands strength, rigidity, inflexibility. Himmler to the SS:

> Most of you here know what it means when 100 corpses lie next to each other, when there are 500 or when there are 1,000. To have endured this and at the same time to have remained a decent person—with exceptions due to human weaknesses—has made us tough, and is a glorious chapter that has not and will not be spoken of.
>
> (Wikipedia, Posen)

The splitting of the ego is self-evident: you can exterminate innocent people and still be a "decent person." Contrary to the typical conflict that Freud describes, here it is morality itself, the imperative to courageously slaughter victims and to remain a "decent," normal person with ordinary human weaknesses, that allows split off, concealed, gratification of macabresque desire.

Weisband uses another aspect of Lacanian theory on this topic. He compares Fonagy on the infant who does not find itself in the mother's mind, but rather the mother herself, to Lacan on the Imaginary. Lacan introduced his idea of the Imaginary in his 1946 paper on the mirror phase. His main idea was that at a certain point in infancy, the baby learns to recognize its own image in the mirror, and is delighted. For Lacan, this is the origin of the narcissistic ego. One sees a reflected *whole* image, and conflates it with oneself. The "split subject of the unconscious" can illusorily be covered over with an intact, undivided image. (Weisband has already cited Bruce Fink on the way *objet a* allows the subject to sustain the illusion of wholeness.) Lacan understands the functioning of the mirror phase as a form of "transitivism," where one attributes one's own actions to the other, as in the child scolded for hitting another child who responds: "I didn't hit him, he hit me." Thus, an early version of accusation in the mirror, of mimetic rivalry. Weisband calls this the "transposed alterity of the Imaginary" (p. 138). One can see the similarity to projective identification, or to the purified pleasure ego. (What

I cannot tolerate about myself is in the other.) Weisband links this process to Segal's symbolic equation and the aggression of the paranoid-schizoid position. He says that blood fantasies "represent savage imaginaries imbued with the fixations of reification that have little or no bearing with 'reality' but serve to embolden perpetrators unable to distinguish object from symbol" (p. 150).

Segal, we have already seen, addresses the ideology of racial differences in just these terms. Weisband, again:

> Beliefs are *concretized* by means of political and social ideologies, or reified forms of language that narcissistically endow human physicality—that is, bodily, skin or corporeal difference in general—with hatred, often in ways parallel to discursive or ideologically constituted forms of political self-adoration
>
> (p. 166; my emphasis)

The political self-adoration is akin to the baby's delight in its apparently intact image. One sees oneself as *not* the racial other. This is another way of conceptualizing how and why the narcissism of racial difference is inevitably violent. But violent in a self-destructive way, greater than childhood transitivism. Once the "split subject of the unconscious" maintains wholeness via mirroring, the subject becomes a "rival self-object unto itself" (p. 138). The paradox being that this results in the "self destructiveness stemming from aggressivity that has been laminated by overlays of narcissist vanity" (p. 155). This is the vanity of the heroic morality described by Himmler. Weisband: "Perpetrators ... envision themselves as acting in the name of personal self-sacrifice while psychically gripped by perverse sadism" (p. 172). *"Performative transgressions punish victims as objects but such punishments are also aimed at perpetrators themselves as their own self-victimizers"* (p. 183; author's emphasis).

Weisband later seems to contradict himself when he returns to Foucault on bio-power: "Sadistic cruelty is not about pleasure but power—the control of the other's body. Victims are to experience the power of another over them" (p. 194).[2] In our discussion of Foucault, we have already tried to demonstrate that his conception of state racism, the "creation" of the "super race" that produces the "sub race," is close to Klein on the paranoid-schizoid position. Weisband has given us the concept of the macabresque, in which the victims' experience of bodily control is a manifestation of the approach to *jouissance*. He has linked this to Lacan on the Imaginary and to Segal on symbolic equation.

Freud himself linked power to sadism and cruelty early on. In *Three Essays on the Theory of Sexuality* (1905), he speaks of what has been translated as an instinct for mastery (in German *Bemächtigungstrieb—macht* can mean power), that is inherently cruel and sadistic:

> the obstacle that brings the instinct for mastery to a halt at another person's pain—namely a capacity for pity—is developed relatively late … It may be assumed that the impulse of cruelty arises from the instinct for mastery.
>
> (1905, p. 193)

In terms of infantile sexuality, this is an aspect of the anal-sadistic phase for Freud. (It would take Klein to explain the late development of a capacity for pity.) Returning to this topic in *Instincts and Their Vicissitudes*, Freud says that at the "stage of the pregenital sadistic-anal organization, the striving for the object appears in the form of an urge for mastery (*Bemächtigungstrieb*), to which injury or annihilation of the object is a matter of indifference. Love in this form and at this preliminary stage is hardly to be distinguished from hate in its attitude towards the object" (1915a, pp. 138–139). This is where Freud proceeds to say that hate as a relation to objects is older than love, and to postulate the purified pleasure ego. If we take "love" in the sexual sense intended by Freud, we can further understand the erotic hatred of the macabresque. Erotic hatred in the service of power, the *Bemächtigungstrieb*—another integration of psychoanalysis and Foucault.

Weisband also engages the question of the legality of genocide. "Sadism is always about the inscriptions of law by extralegal means" (p. 206). For Freud, the origin of law is violence, as in *Totem and Taboo*. In *Thoughts for the Times…*, Freud had said that the state proscribes "wrongdoing" in order to monopolize it, as in war (1915, p. 279). Above, in Kiernan, we cited Major on the divine violence that destroys law. Foucault spoke of the violent inscription of law by extra-legal means. Weisband: "In macabresque sadism, victims must be reduced to the instrumentalities of violation … as a 'right' and 'obligation' bestowed on perpetrators … Perpetrators in the macabresque perform rituals of order, legality, and military command" (p. 206). The ultimate purpose of sadistic, "extralegal" law is control: "The unpredictable and the inconstant, the creative and the 'spontaneous surprise' in human exchange must be brought under control since they become anathema to sadistic aims that detest all forms of singularity and autonomy, difference and otherness" (p. 2026). Bauman called "adiaphoristic action" the fantasized control of unpredictable, "differentiating, and thus potentially divisive, features" (p. 213). The "conceptual Jew," the "foreigner within," embodied the potential uncontrolled division of German identity. Hence, the compulsion to master it, control it, and eliminate it—in the name of the law.

In our discussion of Bauman, we linked the conceptual Jew as threatening difference to the "conceptual Woman," referring to Freud on the strangeness and hostility provoked by sexual difference. Whether the Jew for the Nazis or Woman for Man, the different other becomes "conceptual" in the response to the reality, even the materiality, of difference itself, difference that *cannot* be eliminated, and that *must* be eliminated. The "conceptual" then becomes "concrete," as in Segal's symbolic equation: group beliefs are *"concretized* by means of political and social ideologies, or *reified* forms of language that narcissistically endow human physicality—that is, bodily, skin or corporeal difference in general—with hatred, often in ways parallel to discursive or ideologically constituted forms of political self-adoration" (p. 166; my emphases). Such concretization permits the fantasized possibility of control: you can do something to a material thing, but not to a materiality that is not concrete—difference, otherness. Kiernan, on the Cambodian genocide, said that the actual sight of blood vindicated the idea (i.e., fantasy as "concept") that an infectious agent was being cleansed. He had used the word "fetish" several times. In the introductory chapter, I summarized my own understanding of fetishism: the substitution of opposed fantasies that are taken as *concrete realities,* the defensive substitutes for intolerable difference (e.g., purity and contamination, health and sickness, phallic and castrated in Freud's own concrete version of sexual difference).

This, then, is why perpetrators of genocide, whether a nation or an individual (like Dylann Roof), have to take "the law into their own hands" (p. 207), give themselves the sovereign right to "monopolize violence." There is no more compelling justification for violence than controlling uncontrollable difference. Weisband summarizes what might prevent genocide:

> Subjects must learn to live in the real world of symbolic meanings in which disordered reification reflective of lack, or what Klein called the paranoid-schizoid position, gives ways to distantiation, critical evaluation, and partial acceptance. This is precisely what does not and cannot occur in macabresque sadism
>
> (p. 208)

It was Klein who understood that distantiation, i.e., "withdrawal" of projective identifications, and realization of the "disaster created by one's own sadism," the depressive position, is itself fraught with intense anxieties, always potentially producing regression to the paranoid-schizoid position. When Weisband says that "subjects must learn to live in the real world of symbolic meanings," I take his use of "learn" to mean adapt to, adjust to, accommodate "distantiation"—i.e., difference itself. But what makes that possible? It cannot be "learning" in the cognitive sense, as the affective processes are overwhelmingly intense. Klein already understood this with her postulation of depressive anxieties. To overcome splitting of good and bad, they have to be integrated, but then good might be lost, contaminated by bad. In genocide this is intolerable. Identity collapses if it reintegrates the excluded that constitutes it. Further, the integration of difference, of otherness, is itself a catastrophe, because it threatens the omnipotent control of the uncontrollable. In the clinical situation, the analyst knows that this is an enormous undertaking, potentially traumatizing for the patient, and a great trial for the analyst. Could there be an analogous process on the level of the sovereign nation-state? A process that would enable the state to overcome its concrete fears of contamination? Could there have been any way to counter the Nazi's "conceptual Jew" (Bauman) responsible for uncontrollable chaos?

Notes

1 We referred to Charny on genocide as the "human cancer" in the introduction. We will return to this below.
2 Again, Holslag on power and baby grammar:

> Power over the body is of special importance here. It is, in the most literal sense, the ultimate power one has over another. This power goes further than bureaucratic and institutional power; it is the power over personhood. In this sense violence is the ultimate method of making baby-grammar physical, tangible, visible. (p. 103)

Would Foucault on power over the body be open to thinking of it in terms of baby grammar?

5 Group Phenomena

In the preceding chapter, Weisband cited Kleinian Hanna Segal on groups: "Our psychotic parts are merged into our group identity, and we do not feel mad since our views are sanctioned by the group" (Weisband, p. 157). If the psychosis of genocide is sanctioned by the group, then it is normal. Foucault explained that sovereign power is a function of "real battles, burning towns, ravaged fields and the innocent dead"; its legitimacy "is more basic than any law and is [what] allows laws to function as such" (p. 44). And in relation to both Foucault and Weisband, we referenced Freud in *Totem and Taboo* on the institution of law and society via the murder of the primal father by his sons; if they were to live together, they could not kill each other. In question, then, are the relations of murder, sovereignty, law, and psychosis in groups.

By definition, genocide is always about groups. One group believes it has to protect itself from another group. Even the "lone shooter" is a representative of a group (e.g., Dylann Roof protecting the white race). The group of victims is created through the projective identification of the death drive by the group that believes itself in danger. In genocide the perpetrators' normality is a function of the projective identification of their "psychotic parts" into the victims: "they" madly want to destroy us.

The question of groups and the "normality" of genocide has been especially taken up by James Waller in *Becoming Evil: How Ordinary People Commit Genocide and Mass Killing*. He briefly refers to Freud's *Group Psychology and the Analysis of the Ego* and to the death drive. Freud's book contains an essential analysis of the role of the leader in groups, and also contains the essential passage on the primally violent response to racial difference. The integration of these two topics, via a discussion of *Group Psychology …*, is the prelude to Waller's important analysis of group functioning in genocide.

Freud begins by justifying a psychoanalytic approach to groups:

> If a psychology, concerned with exploring the predispositions, the instinctual impulses, the motives and the aims of an individual man down to his actions and his relations with those who are nearest to him, had

DOI: 10.4324/9781003562870-6

> completely achieved its task, and had cleared up the whole of these matters with their interconnections, it would then suddenly find itself confronted by a new task which would lie before it unachieved. It would be obliged to explain the surprising fact that under a certain condition this individual, whom it had come to understand, thought, felt and acted in quite a different way from what would have been expected. And this condition is his insertion into a collection of people which has acquired the characteristic of a 'psychological group'. What, then, is a 'group'? How does it acquire the capacity for exercising such a decisive influence over the mental life of the individual? And what is the nature of the mental change which it forces upon the individual?
>
> (p. 72)

Here, we can already find hints about the normality of genocide. One might have thoroughly understood the psychodynamics of an individual, and yet find oneself at a loss to explain his unusual behavior in a group. As in Waller's title, ordinary people—with ordinary psychodynamics—can become evil and commit genocide as part of a group.

Freud quotes extensively from Gustave Le Bon's *Psychologie des foules* ("The Psychology of Crowds"). Like Freud, Le Bon says that in a group an individual may act quite differently than in isolation. "There are certain ideas and feelings which do not come into being, or do not transform themselves into acts except in the case of individuals forming a group" (cited, p. 73). Freud agrees, but says that Le Bon does not really explain what makes individuals into a group, i.e., the factor that unites them. Nonetheless, Freud thinks that Le Bon's description of groups "harmonizes well" with psychoanalysis. Le Bon:

> the individual forming part of a group acquires, solely from numerical considerations, a sentiment of invincible power which allows him to yield to instincts which, had he been alone, he would perforce have kept under restraint. He will be the less disposed to check himself, from the consideration that, a group being anonymous and in consequence irresponsible, the sentiment of responsibility which always controls individuals disappears entirely.
>
> (cited, p. 74)

Freud says that Le Bon's "yielding to instincts" which would ordinarily be "kept under restraint" means "throwing off the repressions of drives" (p. 74). This seems self-evident, but Le Bon has also described other themes we have already encountered. He speaks of "invincible power," Foucault's topic *par excellence,* and also the fantasy of invincibility and omnipotence. He says that group anonymity produces irresponsibility, undoing any individual sense of responsibility. For Klein, an individual sense of responsibility arises out of negotiating the depressive position, which means not yielding to the anxieties over integration of good and bad that could produce regression to the paranoid-schizoid position. In the paranoid-schizoid position the only "responsibility"—obligation, really—is to defeat the bad object, and to keep it from contaminating the good object. But we have seen repeatedly that in genocide the obligation to defeat the bad object does become, contra Le Bon, an ethical *responsibility*. ("We had the moral right, we had the duty to our people, to destroy this people which wanted to destroy us.") Diamond called this the combination of instinct and ethics.

Le Bon says that a group is led entirely by "the unconscious," such that its "impulses are always so imperious that no personal interest, not even that of self-preservation, can make itself felt" (cited, p. 77). In other words, what drives a group is so powerful that it overrides the individual, even the individual's self-preservation. *Group Psychology* was published one year after *Beyond the Pleasure Principle*, and we have already seen that Freud does not integrate the theory of the death drive with his analysis of the primally violent response to racial and national difference. Nor does he integrate it with his analysis of groups. (He will allude to *Beyond*... in a footnote.) Nonetheless, when Le Bon speaks of imperious impulses that override individual self-preservation, might one begin to think of a group death drive? An invincible group death drive?

Le Bon: the group

> thinks in images, which call one another up by association (just as they arise with individuals in states of free imagination), and whose agreement with reality is never checked by any reasonable agency. The feelings of a group are always very simple and very exaggerated. So that a group knows neither doubt nor uncertainty
>
> (cited, p. 77)

Freud remarks that this is a description of "unconscious mental life ... as psychoanalysis has long pointed out" (p. 79). Le Bon is basically describing primary process: "thinking" as imagistic, organized by association, unimpeded by "any reasonable agency." This is the usurpation of secondary process by primary process, such that what appears to be thinking is actually fantasizing. As Freud had said about dreams, or in the waking state characterized by delusion or hallucination, there is "neither doubt nor uncertainty." Just as the dream experience feels real, so one cannot argue with a delusion. The implication of Le Bon's passage is that groups can indeed be organized in a psychotic fashion. Thus, he says that

> groups demand illusions, and cannot do without them. They constantly give what is unreal precedence over what is real; they are almost as strongly influenced by what is untrue as by what is true. They have an evident tendency not to distinguish between the two.
>
> (cited, p. 80)

Again, this is a precise description of psychosis, but as per Segal and Le Bon himself, it is normalized by the group. The invincible, omnipotent group.

Le Bon says that groups demand leaders who "make themselves felt by means of the ideas in which they themselves are fanatical believers" (cited, p. 81). The ideas of the leader are the "illusions" (delusions) the group cannot do without. The fanaticism of the leader intensifies the "truth" of the illusion, further normalizing the group psychosis. Freud says that Le Bon does not give an adequate account of the role of the leader, despite "his brilliant description of the group mind" (p. 81). This will be Freud's topic. He summarizes his main point: "*A primary group of this kind is a number of individuals who have put one and the same object in the place of their ego ideal and have consequently identified themselves with one another in their ego*" (p. 116; author's emphasis).

The "ego ideal," as Freud explains, was introduced in his 1914 paper on narcissism (p. 130). There, he spoke of a "differentiating grade" in the ego that is a remnant of original narcissism, i.e., an image of perfection. In *On Narcissism*, he amalgamated this differentiating grade with conscience, such that one part of the ego judges the other for its failure to live up to the idealized image. (This is before the formal introduction of the super-ego in *The Ego and the Id*, 1923.) For Freud, the leader becomes the ego ideal of the group. What holds the group together is the common identification with the leader/ego ideal. Members of the group love each other because they all love the leader.

While Freud does not say so here, in *On Narcissism*, he had spoken about omnipotence as one of the important justifications for studying narcissism, and had linked omnipotence to psychosis. In his concluding remarks about the ego ideal and narcissism in *Group Psychology*, he does say that "when we penetrate deeper into the psychology of the psychoses [the ego ideal's] significance will be discovered to be far greater" (p. 130). What Le Bon called the leader's "fanatical belief" in his ideas can again be understood as the fantasy of omnipotence. Genocide is always an attempt to gain omnipotent control of the uncontrollable. The genocidal leader promises such omnipotence. The shared identification with him is narcissistic, an identification with the promise of omnipotence. For this, one loves the leader.

But groups are not only held together by common identification with an idealized leader. Groups require a sense of "us" that is not "them." Freud adduces this idea casually at first, speaking of the inevitable antipathy between families united by marriage, neighboring towns, etc., such that one group always feels superior to the other (narcissistic grandiosity). But then he goes much further, in the passage about racial difference to which we have alluded several times:

> Closely related races keep one another at arm's length; the South German cannot endure the North German, the Englishman casts every kind of aspersion upon the Scot, the Spaniard despises the Portuguese. We are no longer astonished that greater differences should lead to an almost

> insuperable repugnance, such as the Gallic people feel for the German, the Aryan for the Semite, and the white races for the coloured [...] In the undisguised antipathies and aversions which people feel towards strangers with whom they have to do we may recognize the expression of self-love—of narcissism. This self-love works for the preservation of the individual, and behaves as though the occurrence of any divergence from his own particular lines of development involved a criticism of them and a demand for their alteration. We do not know why such sensitiveness should have been directed to just these details of differentiation; but it is unmistakable that in this whole connection men give evidence of a readiness for hatred, an aggressiveness, the source of which is unknown, and to which one is tempted to ascribe an elementary character.
>
> (pp. 101–102)

At the end of this passage, Freud appends a footnote: "In a recently published study, *Beyond the Pleasure Principle,* I have attempted to connect the polarity of love and hatred with a hypothetical opposition between instincts of life and death" (note 1, p. 102).

It is somewhat astonishing that Freud simply mentions *Beyond...* here, and does not employ his theorization of life and death to understand the "unknown" "elementary character" of the narcissistic hatred of the different other. Freud is clear in *Beyond...* that the life drive introduces "fresh vital differences" into the psyche, thereby raising tension levels. He is equally clear that the death drive, like the pleasure principle, reduces tension, and that self-destruction is projected outward in the form of sadism and hatred. And we have seen that "hate as a relation to objects is older than love," because the pleasure principle demands projection outward of any intolerable internal tension, producing the purified pleasure ego. We can now say that the purified pleasure ego is narcissistic: all good is in me, what is other is not good—because it embodies my projected badness. Racial and/or national groups, defined by what they are not, are a kind of *purified pleasure group*. A group united by its love for the promise of narcissistic omnipotence provided by the leader. In genocide, this results in not only the normalization, but also the glorification, the idealization of destruction of the racial/national other.

In *On Narcissism,* while the ego ideal was amalgamated with conscience, there was no mention of the Oedipus complex and guilt. In *The Ego and the Id,* Freud extends his understanding of the ego ideal, renaming it the superego. Now, Freud integrates several strands of his theory. When we have to give up a libidinal object, we tend to identify with it. The Oedipus complex places this demand on the child. But the identification with the Oedipal objects is a reaction formation against them, and thus a kind of negative image of the investment in them.

> By setting up this ego ideal, the ego has mastered the Oedipus complex and at the same time placed itself in subjection to the id. Whereas the ego

> is essentially the representative of the external world, of reality, the super-ego stands in contrast to it as the representative of the internal world, of the id.
>
> (1923, p. 36)

On one hand, as the expansion of the ego ideal, the super-ego is the embodiment of conscience, judging the ego for its id wishes, creating guilt. On the other, as a reaction formation against the id, the super-ego's energy comes from the id.

Because the super-ego borrows its energy from the id, its morality is sadistic, id like:

> How is it that the super-ego manifests itself essentially as a sense of guilt (or rather, as criticism—for the sense of guilt is the perception in the ego answering to this criticism) and moreover develops such extraordinary harshness and severity towards the ego? If we turn to melancholia first, we find that the excessively strong super-ego which has obtained a hold upon consciousness rages against the ego with merciless violence, as if it had taken possession of the whole of the sadism available in the person concerned. Following our view of sadism, we should say that the destructive component had entrenched itself in the super-ego and turned against the ego. What is now holding sway in the super-ego is, as it were, a pure culture of the death instinct, and in fact it often enough succeeds in driving the ego into death [...] it may be said of the id that it is totally non-moral, of the ego that it strives to be moral, and of the super-ego that it can be super-moral and then become as cruel as only the id can be.
>
> (pp. 53–54)

When Freud says that in melancholia (depression) the super-ego has "taken possession of the whole of the sadism available in the person concerned," such that it is a "pure culture of the death instinct," there is a sense in which he is echoing Melanie Klein on the origin of the super-ego. In the paranoid-schizoid position, there is mandatory projection of the death drive, creating the persecutory bad object, and then incorporation of this bad object, a re-introjection of the death drive. For Klein, this explains what Freud describes here in terms of melancholia: the formation of an internal object that sadistically, destructively attacks the ego. This is why Klein calls this internal persecutor the origin of the super-ego. One might see it as the oral and anal phase precursors of Freud's Oedipal super-ego.

Let us return to group dynamics in genocide. We have spoken of a "purified pleasure group," on the model of Freud's purified pleasure ego. The latter has a relation to Klein on projective identification: what is bad in me is in the other, the original hatred of the object. The primal urge to destroy the different other is justified by the delusional belief that the group of different others wants to destroy "us," a possibility that Freud did not imagine, but which

Klein could explain. Whatever guilt "we" might feel for our destructiveness is projected into "them": *they* are guilty of their wish to destroy *us* ("this people who want to destroy us"). Or perhaps not even guilty: like a virus, they have to infect and attack us. The leader is fanatically certain of this. The "purified pleasure" group is held together by identification with this idealized figure. In genocide, this idealized figure embodies both the primal wish to destroy the different others *and* the mechanisms of the paranoid-schizoid position. *The genocidal group is united in identification with the idealized paranoid-schizoid position of the leader as omnipotent good object, whose id-based fantasies make the victims into persecutors and holds the group together.* As per Klein, where there is idealization (a good object) there is always persecutory anxiety (a bad object). Since "they" are guilty, they occupy the position Freud described for the ego in melancholia; they are raged against with "merciless violence." A violence that becomes law and morality themselves, the sadistic super-ego as a "pure culture of the death instinct." A narcissistically idealized, omnipotent, merciless, *sovereign* right to kill.

The title of Waller's book seems to emphasize the individual and the perennial question of "how ordinary people commit genocide." But he is perfectly aware that group dynamics are a crucial part of the explanation. In his introduction, he says that "we engage in acts of extraordinary evil, with apparent moral calm and intensity of purpose, which could only be considered as insane were they committed by an individual" (p. xv). He is already suggesting that group dynamics can produce a "normal psychosis" that is morality itself. And he says that "If we use the number of deaths as the basis for assigning importance, it can be argued that there is no more pressing problem facing humans today" (p. xvi). Nor is he blind to the evolutionary aspect of the question: "Can it be abnormal despite its constant presence within our species?" (p. 8). Later in the book, looking at "us/them" thinking from an evolutionary perspective, he cites the research on "xenophobic" chimps (pp. 184–185) that Diamond also used. The problem is that while "pro-social" adaptation, i.e., living in groups, has been crucial to the success of *Homo sapiens*, hurting those in other groups can be selectively advantageous (p. 158). "Group selection favors within-group niceness *and* between-group nastiness" (p. 158). This is a "hereditary dark side that is universal across humankind" (p. 158).

Waller agrees with Le Bon that whoever supplies the group with illusions is their master; whoever tries to destroy illusions is their victim (p. 33). And he agrees with Freud's extensions of Le Bon, namely that groups are dominated by the unconscious, the id; and that the super-ego is transferred to the leader (pp. 34–35). Once the leader's conscience sanctions violence, individuals are free to do the same. Sounding like Foucault, Waller says that collectives respond to, and are dislodged by, only one thing—power (p. 36).

But groups are not in and of themselves violent or evil. They can develop practices and values that promote care and connection. Ultimately, the nature of the group depends upon the individuals within it. "There is psychological continuity between individuals and the group" (p. 40). This continuity itself reflects "human nature": it is uncomfortable to admit that culture or ideology are the "pretexts" for the more general wish to dominate and destroy, which are "universal aspects of human nature" (p. 53), the "hereditary dark side that is universal across humankind." Evolution, natural selection itself, Waller thinks, has not been "as efficient in crafting adaptations on the group level as it is on the individual level" (p. 157). In other words, while "hurting those in other groups can be selectively advantageous," the propensity to dominate and destroy can also produce potentially nonadaptive group behavior. "No other species shows the degree of mass killings of its own species that humans do" (p. 161). This fact compels us to think of *Homo sapiens* itself as a murderously self-destructive group. When Foucault called Nazi Germany "an absolutely racist state, an absolutely murderous state, and an absolutely suicidal state" he perhaps did not imagine that one might substitute "species" for (Nazi) "state" in his description.

This large group reasoning makes Waller oppose the delineation of any particular personality type to explain genocide. He thinks that Adorno's study of the authoritarian personality, for example, "tells us more about our own personal dreams of how we wish the world to work than it does about perpetrator behavior. In that role, such explanations satisfy an important emotional demand of distancing *us* from *them*" (p. 91, author's emphasis). In other words, confining genocide to a particular personality organization is another manifestation of us/them group behavior. "Our" personality organization is not like "theirs." Since there have always been those who recognize and oppose genocide, one might imagine this to be a simple truth. But if the ability to take responsibility for one's aggression, to overcome the splitting into good and bad, is a manifestation of Klein's depressive position, consciously or unconsciously there has been a grappling with the paranoid-schizoid potential in everyone. This would also make it possible *not* to succumb to the primal wish to destroy difference. To confine genocidal behavior to "them" is not only to betray a wish for how the world would work, but also a wish for how the mind of *Homo sapiens might* work.

On this question of the wish for how the mind might work, Waller inevitably encounters Freud on the death drive. He gives a quick overview of Freud on drives, from the original emphasis on sexuality, through self-preservation, to aggression and destructiveness. Waller correctly notes that the postulation of a death drive to explain destructiveness was in part derived from Freud's reaction to World War I *and* from the compulsion to repeat "self defeating or painful acts" (p. 145). The death drive then became "an innate universal urge across humankind" that encompassed "all impulses toward hostility, sadism, aggression" and even "a mysterious drive toward one's own death" (p 145). Waller agrees with the many who reject "Freud's specific concept of a death instinct," while accepting that "human nature has a tendency toward aggression" (p. 146). "Recognizing that aggression can be closely linked with self-preservation and self-affirmation reminds us that it need not be derived from a 'death instinct'" (p. 146). This is where Waller himself might be wishing for a model of how the mind might work. What he does not consider, is the paradox of self-defeating, self-destructive self-preservation. This is the universal tendency of *Homo sapiens* to create a "purified pleasure *group*" in thrall to an idealized paranoid-schizoid leader who glorifies hatred of those who contain his own projected self-destructiveness.

Waller emphasizes that when "group membership is seen as impermeable and fixed, the potential to view other groups as perpetual threats is heightened" (p. 174). We have already encountered the question of impermeable boundaries in Bauman: what is foreign is not supposed to be inside. But the "foreign body" is a creation of the very "body" it is not supposed to be inside (the autoimmune response; Foucault's superrace creating its own subrace). Thus, the wish for the impermeable boundary is a manifestation of its threatening permeability, porousness. "Impermeable and fixed" group membership is under "perpetual threat." As the threat increases so does the violence the group imagines is necessary. And so does the fantasy that every one of "them" is identical and "interchangeable" (p. 174). Each one of them is identically opposed to "us," is the "bad" contrary of our "goodness." If "we" do not understand this, "we" foolishly leave ourselves open to destruction. The more "we" use collective violence to kill the foreigner within, the more "in-group solidarity" is enhanced. This solidarity itself enhances "our" goodness: we are purified.

Waller adduces the familiar question of the role of religion:

> religious belief systems emphasizing divine influence and authority may be particularly relevant in shaping our responses to *worldly* influence and authority [...] Just as religious belief systems are an element in the impulse to heal, they also can be an element in the impulse to kill [...] Most religious belief systems are [...] ethnocentric and [...] may even foster a devaluing effect on the human life that falls outside the veil of the faithful. They distinguish all too clearly between 'us' and 'them,' [...] between those whom the gods love and those whom they hate.
>
> (p. 182; author's emphasis)

In the chapter on Kiernan, we have seen the historical importance of the Old Testament genocides against the Midianites and the Amalakites, hated by the one, true god. The "worldly influence" Waller speaks of is the translation of murder into ethical imperative, what Rene Major called "divine violence": "the mythical violence that attempts to found the right to a new order needs to depend upon divine violence to establish the justice of its cause, a violence irreducible to law, a violence that destroys law" (1999, p. 142). Note that Major speaks of a "justice" that "destroys law." This sounds oxymoronic, but is precisely the point. Once violence is divinely enjoined it destroys its own law: "thou shalt not kill" becomes "thou shalt kill in my name those

I deem evil." Divinity becomes the leader of the leader, whether the leader is manifestly religious or not.[1]

Waller grounds us/them collective group identities in ethnocentrism and xenophobia. He sees these too as "ultimate, universal human tendencies" from our "evolutionary heritage" (p. 199)—chimp xenophobia. Both have their roots in "caretaker-infant bonds and stranger anxiety of the first year of life" (p. 200). Recall Holslag on "baby grammar." Hence, "the evolution of sociability, altruism, and cooperation goes hand in hand with the evolution of animosity to outsiders" (p. 200). Waller cites Ghiglieri:

> Xenophobia and ethnocentrism are not just essential ingredients to war. Because they instinctively tell men precisely whom to bond with versus whom to fight against, they are the most dangerously manipulable facets of war psychology that promote genocide. Indeed, genocide itself has become a potent force in human evolution.
>
> (cited, p. 201)

But there is more to it than that. The threatened group identity that promotes genocide, the "perpetrators' sense of vulnerability," "comes easily from the part of our psyche that wants to view ourselves as victims or potential victims" (p. 205). Clearly, Waller is now speaking of not only ethnocentrism and xenophobia grounded in the mother–infant bond and stranger anxiety, but also of masochism.

No one saw more clearly than Freud the interchangeability of sadism and masochism. To recapitulate what was outlined above in Weisband: in *Instincts and Their Vicissitudes*, Freud accounted for interchangeable sadism and masochism with a postulated primary "intermediate" phase out of which the active and passive forms of pleasure in pain arise. Later, in *The Economic Problem of Masochism*, he postulated primary masochism, due to the portion of the death drive that remains within the organism and is fused with libido. Hence, where there is masochism there is also sadism, which Waller examines in a chapter on "The Social Construction of Cruelty." He necessarily refers to the famous experiments of Milgram and Zimbardo. (The first, at Yale, found that subjects were willing to administer what they were led to believe were powerfully painful electric shocks to invisible subjects; the second, at Stanford, created an artificial prison situation in which "guards" began to act so sadistically that the experiment had to be stopped.) Both Milgram and Zimbardo stress context, "situation." Zimbardo: "Individual behavior is largely under the control of social forces and environmental contingencies rather than personality traits, character, will power or other empirically unvalidated constructs" (cited, p. 231). Milgram:

> Many people, not knowing about the experiment [obedience to authority], claim that subjects who go to the end of the board [of electric shocks]

> are sadistic. Nothing could be more foolish [...] The context of action must always be considered. The individual, upon entering the laboratory, becomes integrated into a situation that carries its own momentum
> (cited, p. 231)

Weisband's study of the "macabresque" nonetheless found that cruelty for its own sake always accompanies genocide. Waller considers both factors: the relation of sadism to group behavior and the social construction of cruelty.

Waller's basic point is that "Perpetrators create, and are created by, a social construction of cruelty ... Such a context of cruelty makes each perpetrator believe that all are capable of doing what he or she does" (p. 231). Clearly Waller finds an interaction of both active and passive behaviors—"create, and are created by." Going back to Le Bon and Freud on the leader's "fanatical" belief in his illusions; on the liberation of repressed drives in groups, and on the basic idea of strength in numbers; Waller is vindicating *both* the influence of context *and* the unleashing of a sadistic potential. The perpetrator is not wrong to "believe" that many, if not all, are "capable of doing what he or she does." As we saw in the chapter on Kiernan, this is why "accusation in the mirror" works. Hence, the interaction of active and passive between the leader and the group. What Milligram and Zimbardo are perhaps unwilling to recognize is that their subjects could have had a sadistic potential unleashed in a particular context, and then return to ordinary functioning, as in the entire history of genocide.

Waller analyzes this process in terms of "escalating commitments": "... an initial, relatively inconsequential, evil act can make later evildoing easier. Once one has taken the initial step, one is in a new social context in which the pressures to continue are quite powerful" (p. 232). He cites the research of Janice Gibson and Mika Haritos-Fatouros on the gradual, systematic training of torturers under the Greek military dictatorship (1967–1974). They were initially subject to abuse and torture themselves, while being told "how fortunate they were to be invited into such an elite organization" (p. 233)—a narcissistic idealization of masochism. They then became willing torturers—sadism. Gibson and Haritos "found no evidence of sadistic, abusive, or authoritarian behavior in the Greek soldiers' histories prior to their training" (p. 233), meaning no conscious evidence. When journalist Gitta Sereny asked Franz Stangl, commandant of Treblinka, why the killing of the Jews was organized so as to achieve the maximum humiliation of victims, he replied: "To condition those who actually had to carry out the policies. To make it possible for them to do what they did" (p. 234). This is another confirmation of Weisband's thesis about the "macabresque," and its usefulness for creating the group dynamics of genocide. Waller puts this as a question that is really a statement: "Could it be that as we work our way into a context of cruelty, the cruelty also works its way into us?" (p. 235). Despite Zimbardo's emphasis on context, on "good apples in bad barrels" (cited, p. 238), even he says about the prison experiment: "Most dramatic and distressing to us, was the observation of the ease with which sadistic behavior could be elicited in individuals who were not 'sadistic types' " (cited, p. 237).

Waller cites research that seems to disconfirm the relation between sadism and group dynamics. There are many accounts of the Nazi soldiers who participated in genocide having to get drunk to carry out their work, or even committing suicide (p. 245). There are equally accounts of desensitization, of perpetrators initially horrified by their work, but for whom it became routine (p. 237). Nonetheless, research also confirms, as Weisband theorized, that there is always a small number of openly sadistic perpetrators who enjoy their work, for whom there is an "almost addiction-like quest for pleasure" (citied, p. 246). There are individual testimonies of perpetrators who found killing as pleasurable as sex (p. 246). Even if their numbers are initially small, the unleashing of this potential in genocide does support the idea of sado-masochistic dynamics in the "purified pleasure group." Waller thinks that "our external behaviors and roles so dramatically affect our internal psychological framework," because

> we tend toward integration between the external and the internal [...] we are troubled by inconsistencies between *what* we do and *who* we think we are. We are motivated to alleviate these inconsistencies to preserve the integrity of the self.
>
> (p. 239)

When context is a (divinely) sovereign state with the right, or even ethical obligation, to kill, the "context of cruelty works it way into us." Returning to Waller's statement about the "psychological continuity between individuals and the group," it is essential to remember that the creation of context itself depends upon the unconscious dynamics in individuals. Which is why "We cannot, and should not, displace responsibility to the situation rather than the person" (p. 269).

This is obviously the justification for the trials of perpetrators, from Nuremberg to Dylann Roof. Such trials must take place. However, focusing exclusively on the individual leaves the "situation" untouched. Can one try a "context," a group, a nation?[2] It has often been said that nations do not have consciences. Indeed, "the harsh reality is that most states lack the will to enlarge their definition of national interest to include the prevention, stopping, or punishing of genocide" (p. 281). Perhaps this is putting it too mildly once sovereignty is the right to kill. From the small groups of neighbors and families to the larger groups of nations that Freud spoke of, the maintenance of an identity that is *not them*, inevitably links the group to what we call "race," and the violent response to it—which Freud also spoke of. Genocide becomes the "national interest." Waller says that "We must persist in our pursuit of a greater 'us.' To not do so is to fall prey to our evolutionarily primed tendencies of ethnocentrism and xenophobia" (p. 291). But this means that this evolution is installed in the sovereign nation-state, our unquestioned contemporary form of government, just as it is in our unconscious dynamics. Does this lead to an almost unthinkable question: to prevent genocide, must *Homo sapiens* take on responsibility for its own evolution? Is something like this imaginable?

Notes

1 This is the theme of the theology of sovereignty which Derrida will take up. See below.

2 The International Criminal Court can try *individuals* for such crimes as genocide and mass murder, and has done so. However, not all nations are signatories of the court, including the United States. The International Court of Justice can hear cases brought by one *nation* against another for similar crimes.

6 The Cancer Metaphor

Israel Charny is an Israeli psychologist who did his undergraduate and graduate degrees in the United States. He has written a great deal on the Holocaust and genocide. His psychological approach and many references to psychoanalytic theory integrates much of what has preceded here. The title of his book summarizes the essential problem: *How Can We Commit the Unthinkable?* His subtitle hints at what is original in his approach: *Genocide: The Human Cancer*.

In his introduction, Charny says that his "theme-metaphor" is "destructiveness as a cancer like process that, like physical cancer, is latent in all of us" (p. xiii). Explaining a bit more, he says that potentially lethal cancer cells are "always present in the human organism. In states of disease, the process of life is somehow overwhelmed by these ever-present cancer cells, which previously were held in balance by the larger life system" (p. 33). What unbalances the "larger life system" such that cancer overwhelms the organism? The "organism" here being the "combination of personal and collective forces that can explain the evils of genocide" (p. 24).

Charny's position is akin to Freud's and Waller's on the continuity between the individual and the group. He too, wants to understand man's "madness of destruction and genocide" via "everyday hurts and hurting others" (p. 2). But he also sees genocide as "a total configuration of events that is determined on many levels of political, economic, and sociological forces acting through the barely understood power of the group process on an individual human nature we know too little about" (p. 4).

Like Waller and Diamond the "group" Charny imagines is *Homo sapiens*. That genocide is the *human* cancer, indicates that "man is at a primitive point in his evolution" (p. 21). Later he cites Konrad Lorenz on the idea that most animals do not commit extensive violence to members of their own species (p. 190). (Although recall "xenophobic chimps"). "For Lorenz, the fact that human beings do not follow this rule is a disturbing indication that something has gone wrong in man's very evolution" (p. 190). Thus, the perhaps impossible question raised at the end of the chapter on Waller: can man take charge of his own evolution? Charny, in fact, sees this as a real possibility: "…

DOI: 10.4324/9781003562870-7

it is in the very nature of the same evolutionary process that man represents the emergence of a fuller consciousness that allows him to choose and direct much of the subsequent thrust of his own evolution" (p. 94).

But even Charny's own discipline shows evidence of the evolutionary problem:

> It is hard to tell yet whether there is a truly deep concern over the bedrock destructiveness of the 'normal' human being, for even now, psychology books rarely contain an honest description of how the normal personality includes an explicit penchant for destructiveness.
>
> (p. 20)

(Perhaps true of "psychology books," but not of psychoanalysis. Recall Freud on the primal hatred that abhors and attempts to destroy; Klein on the mechanisms of the paranoid-schizoid position; and Weisband's use of psychoanalytic theory to explain the "macabresque.") The general marginalization of psychoanalysis is itself a manifestation of the evolutionary problem. Charny cites McNeil: "Man's psychic nature cannot remain an unknown in the equation of violence, or we will find ourselves presiding over the dissolution of the human race" (cited, p. 27).

Charny's understanding of the action of the human cancer depends upon his model of "psycho-atomic energy" (p. 48). While one might pause at the term "psycho-atomic," Charny is analogizing basic physical forces to psychic forces. There is a "basic interplay or polarization of positive and negative forces. Energy is then generated from the impact of creating elements and building elements poised in counterpoint against forces for tearing down and breaking down" (p. 48). This sounds very much like the Freud of *Beyond the Pleasure Principle,* who spoke about life and death as "assimilatory" and "dissimilatory" forces (1920. p. 49). Freud later compared love and hate to the "polarity of attraction and repulsion that plays a part in your [Einstein's] own field of knowledge" (1933, p. 209); and to pre-Socratic philosopher Empedocles' conception that *philia* (love) and *neikos* (strife) are the two great forces in the universe (1937, p. 246). Charny uses another analogy: "the biologist's conception of anabolic or life-building processes and catabolic or breaking-down forces" (p. 50). Freud gives a slightly more complex version of the same analogy. Speaking of the life and death drives, he says: "a special physiological process (of anabolism or catabolism) would be associated with each of the two classes of instincts" (1923, p. 41).

Charny combines his energetic idea with the problem of evolution:

> in our current stage of human evolution, individually and collectively, we frequently do not succeed in marshaling a balanced controlled flow of energy. All too often, humankind explodes in madness. In the metaphor, I propose to think of such madness as failures to balance out the positive building and the negative, tearing down components [...] when

> a significant excess of either the positive or the negative force develops, there is compensatory activity on the part of the opposite or complementary force.
>
> (p. 53)

In a similar vein, Freud says:

> It is as though the life of the organism moved with a vacillating rhythm. One group of instincts rushes forward so as to reach the final aim of life as swiftly as possible [death]; but when a particular stage in the advance has been reached, the other group jerks back to a certain point to make a fresh start [life].
>
> (1920, pp. 40–41)

This relation of evolution to considerations of energy is critical to understanding the relation of the individual and the collective in genocide. When a group idealizes a leader who promotes the destructiveness of the paranoid-schizoid position, there is a simultaneous increase of "positive" and "negative" force within the group, and "negative" force outside the group. As Freud had said, there is an anabolic and catabolic aspect to each of the two forces. Within the genocidal group, the negative force projected onto the victims consolidates the positive force within the group, but also consolidates the self-destructive force within the group. Returning to Freud on the super-ego and the death drive, and to the analogy of the relation of the genocidal group to melancholia: "...the excessively strong super-ego which has obtained a hold upon consciousness rages against the ego with merciless violence ... What is now holding sway in the super-ego is, as it were, a pure culture of the death instinct" (1923, p. 53). In other words, the leader as the ego ideal/super-ego of the group unleashes the collective force of the destructiveness (the "cancer") inherent in the individual and does so as a glorified ethical principle, promising omnipotence. The "explosion" of madness Charny describes is normalized by the intensification of "attraction" in the group, and the erotization of self-destructiveness, akin to what Freud called primary masochism. Weisband's use of Lacan's *jouissance* to understand the "macabresque" makes an analogous point.

Thus, Charny makes the simple, but not self-evident, argument that the most important indicator of psychopathology is "respect for human life ... and respect for the integrity of the lives of others" (p. 17). In Kleinian terms, such "inner integrity" (p. 17) depends upon negotiation of the depressive position. But when the "power of the group" only respects the integrity of the lives of those within the group, the mechanisms of the paranoid-schizoid position are normalized, and even idealized. Charny similarly notes: "Man's gods freely call for death to man's enemies even as the gods preach the injunction 'Thou shalt not kill'" (p. 25). Hence, the "divine violence" that is more basic than law, and that institutes law (Major), such that genocide can be an ethical command. To bring about the death of others makes one nearly divine, proving one's "own omnipotence," one's "control" over "life and death" (p. 44). Recall Foucault on populations, on the power to decide who lives and who dies.

This leads Charny to describe another kind of "normal psychosis":

> We certainly know a good deal about how people who are lacking in loving may be deeply destructive, but it is too easy a matter to dismiss such people as simply angry and hence destructive. Often there is a terrible unknowing ache of emptiness, and a wish for contact and love that feels so unreachable, that these lonely souls are driven to power- and destruction-seeking fantasies and acts as ways to express themselves, feel alive, and gain contact—any kind of contact— with others. *These lonely souls have been known to put on the gray shirts and brown shirts and black boots of their respective eras and bash people's brains in.*
>
> (p. 57; author's emphasis)

This might certainly be the profile of individuals whose lives are fulfilled by joining the genocidal group.[1] However, we also know that those who put on the gray and brown shirts might be apparently normal people who are not such "lonely souls." But, what if they feel *most* alive, *most* in contact with others, when they bash in the brains of those who "threaten" the existence of the group? What if their *esprit de corps* is intensified not only by destructiveness, but also by the collective submission to the *love* of the "pure culture of the death instinct" of the leader? Charny speaks of "false feelings of aliveness through destructiveness" (p. 86), having already said that "People who are destructive of others generally wind up destroyed" (p. 61).

This is where Charny takes up the Foucauldian theme of power. He says that there

> can be a great deal of pleasure in the discovery that one has achieved power over others, there can be delight at the apparent confirmation of oneself as strong, and there can be gratification in finding long-standing fantasies and wishes to control others coming true.
>
> (p. 65)

Foucault would probably reject this psychological account of power, given his theory of power as something that circulates. But that is not so far from Charny on the relation of power to distributions of energy:

> there is much we do not know about how to store, transmit, and channel our power [...] it is in the nature of power—when expressed or directed toward others —to press, penetrate, and ultimately attack, hurt, and fell. It is in the nature of power to be what it is by virtue of nothing more than the momentum of the thrust of energy [...] It is also in the nature of power

> to be destructive of another when the other person is unable to stand up against the energy directed at him.
>
> (p. 64)

Above we juxtaposed Foucault on the "creation" of the "subrace" out of the "superrace" with Klein on splitting. The way in which the idealization of the leader's paranoid-schizoid "fantasies and wishes" promises omnipotence, power, and control to the group intensifies the love for the leader and the group; this love is further intensified by the pleasure in achieving the power to destroy others. Freud had already cited Le Bon on the "sentiment of invincible power" in groups, which allows the individual to "yield to instincts" which he otherwise would have been restrained. Waller said that groups respond to only one thing—power, and referenced those perpetrators who found "killing as pleasurable as sex."

When Weisband spoke of the "noir ecstasy" of the macabresque, he too understood it as allowing "perpetrators to revel in their absolute power" (p. 99), as the result of the projection of unbearable shame and humiliation onto victims, who then become objects of revenge and revulsion (p. 10). Charny has a similar analysis:

> Another side to the gratifications yielded by power over others derives from our always lurking need to project our most feared weaknesses onto others [...] the machinery of the human mind tries to put on others those qualities we are most unhappy about in ourselves, and most fear for ourselves. It takes considerable emotional growth to learn to forgo the natural temptation to attribute to others those parts of ourselves that we can't stand. It seems almost beyond human nature to expect people not to take advantage of opportunities for control over others [...] 'Here is somebody on whom I can put what I can't stand in myself. I would be mad to pass this opportunity by'.
>
> (pp. 65–66)

Again we are reminded of Freud's purified pleasure ego which unreservedly "hates, abhors, and seeks to destroy" the objects which have been created by projection of what is unbearable in oneself; of Klein on projective identification; and of Holslag's "reverse mirroring" and "baby grammar."

Not only would it be mad to forgo the opportunity to rid oneself of the unbearable via projection (or projective identification), it is even madder not to protect ourselves against such objects, who are obviously out to destroy us. Charny also reaches this conclusion. Once a given group has been "dehumanized" by projection:

> we also need to 'prove' that they are out to hurt us [...], proof that the others are also a terrible threat to our lives and that it is their intent to take our lives away from us unless we stop them first [...] First we project our

> feared weakness onto the others, then we project our destructive murderous impulses onto them, and most of all what we project onto the hapless target group is that they are to be the object of the death we so fear for ourselves [...] it is entirely justified that we destroy them.
>
> (p. 109)

The result is the "mad spectacle" of *Homo sapiens,*

> a brilliantly evolving organism that is making breathtaking penetrations into the secrets of nature, extending life, and building fascinating and beautiful civilizations on the one hand and on the other, given to simple minded, primitive magic-ridden devices to create and maintain illusions, self deception, and actual psychotic delusions to protect itself from terror.
>
> (p. 106)

Again, psychology itself has not measured up to this reality, has not dealt with the "...universality of various *bizarre psychic processes*, which psychological theory has not effectively encompassed in its overall picture of *normal* man" (p. 88; my emphases).

Such bizarre processes often depend upon "dehumanization." This can explain why *Homo sapiens* can commit mass violence against members of its own species; it psychotically believes that these are *not* members of its own species. Charny explains this as a function of the "group life" in which "the mechanism of projection seizes on the differences between people. From the very beginning of life, human beings are aware of the difference between the strange and the familiar" (p. 188). The familiar is the mother, but there is "considerable anxiety about the loss of the mother. The process of handling separation anxiety is one of the critical processes in an infant's early development" (p. 188). The different other then embodies what is strange, and is the inevitable target of projection:

> The stranger [...] represents all of people's fears of aloneness, vulnerability, and ultimate death [...] it takes a considerable amount of experience to learn to trust those are very different from us and to experience our common humanity with them [...] if people who are very different from us are slaughtered, we are not likely to have any sense of emotional involvement.
>
> (p. 189)

Charny outlines the process that leads from stranger anxiety to dehumanization, based upon the "awareness of difference" (p. 190). At first, this may be a question of familiarity: one is not comfortable with those who are different. This "level of projection" can "escalate" to the point of seeing "other people as less valuable" (p. 190). The less valuable may then be seen as "not of our kind ... even not of our species" (p. 190). This "sets the stage for possible violence to them" (p. 190). War and genocide cannot possibly end "unless and until we have tools for containing projection processes" (p. 190). In his own way, Charny here rejoins Freud on the narcissistically violent response to national and racial difference from *Group Psychology*. Above, in relation to Bauman on the "conceptual Jew," we also looked at Freud on what we called the "conceptual woman," the woman who is other than man, and thus strange, unfamiliar, and uncanny. Ultimately, it is a question of every variation on the defensive response to difference.

The aim is the "flux of differences," which "provides a better basis for stability than any imposition of a rigid pattern of sameness" (p. 83). "The metaphor of good and bad as intertwined is consistent with ... the cultural process that speak[s] to the vitality ... of those social systems that include unsettled, changing, vital processes of conflicts, differences" (p. 82). Destructiveness often imposes "order and sameness on everything," in order to "remove the dangers of spontaneity and naturalness" (p. 83). Weisband: "The unpredictable and the inconstant, the creative and the 'spontaneous surprise' in human exchange must be brought under control since they become anathema to sadistic aims that detest all forms of singularity and autonomy, difference and otherness" (p. 206). The paradox of these statements is that what one might call the "instability" of difference actually stabilizes life, is vital.

All of which calls for further integration of Freud and Klein on difference and good and bad "intertwined." Charny has already spoken of the "psychoatomic" forces of building and destroying, very much akin to what Freud has said about the life and death drives. He explicitly refers to "the epic work of Freud" (p. 68) on this topic, but offers a shift in emphasis:

> In Freud, generally, Eros and Thanatos are joined in a death struggle of the gods, and only one can win. Freud emphasizes not so much the value of uniting both good and evil aspects of life, but the energy that comes from choosing building over tearing down, or the affirmation of life over the taking away of life. The opposing forces of creating and destroying are posed essentially as antagonistic to one another more than as two sides of our humanness working together
>
> (p. 68)

This is not quite right. Above we cited Freud to the effect that "a special physiological process (of anabolism or catabolism) would be associated with each of the two classes of instincts" (1920, p. 41). Precisely for this reason, Freud is clear that the life drive introduces "fresh vital differences" into the organism, which is simultaneously catabolistic (differentiation breaks down) and anabolistic (it integrates with what is other). For this reason too, Freud is clear that the life drive increases "vitality," raising the tension levels in the organism, but will always be met by the dedifferentiating, tension-reducing death drive, "the struggle against Eros." There is always a kind of antilife autoimmune process in life itself, perhaps what Charny means by his cancer metaphor.

The reference to the "intertwining" of good and bad has to recall Klein on the paranoid-schizoid and depressive positions. The former projects the death drive, creating the bad object, and then splits the idealized good and the persecutory bad objects. The latter integrates them, but is necessarily prey to anxieties over loss of the good object when it is "contaminated" by the bad. This, in fact, would be another facet of separation and stranger anxiety—the catastrophic loss of the familiar, good object when it becomes "unfamiliar," bad, strange. This is why Klein says that depressive anxiety over integration can produce regression to paranoid-schizoid mechanisms, which, in Freud's terms, means exacerbation of the working of the death drive. In *The Ego and the Id* (1923), Freud made what he called a "swift generalization" when he characterized regression as a "defusion of instincts," i.e. an increasing dominance of the death drive (p. 42). This is why we have emphasized that when the leader of a group promotes the "normal psychosis" of the paranoid-schizoid position, he becomes an idealized, omnipotent figure, promoting love within the group, and hatred outside it, the kind of drive defusion Freud described.

The critical integration of Freud and Klein here is that since life, vitality itself, requires integration with difference as tension, it can always be countered by the death drive. Splitting then will have it that difference is the opposition of good and bad. The different other as a narcissistic threat becomes something entirely other, not even of "our" own species. Thus, Charny says that "it is difficult, even far fetched, to hope for a control of processes like projection and dehumanization on the broad plane of international relations" (p. 209). More emphatically:

> The correspondence between Klein's picture of the basic emotional interaction between the child and its mother and the ways in which people and nations behave toward one another on far more complex levels of interaction is, to say the least, impressive.
>
> (p. 246)

Pursuing the cancer metaphor to its logical conclusion, Charny says that once genocide is underway, "the cancer cannot be stopped, of course, except by destroying the host" (p. 316). Genocide itself speaks to the "universal latent impulse to erupt in mad, defiant, omnipotent-seeking rage (that is often at the same time a covert prelude to rest or suicide)" (p. 227). The death drive is the ultimate dedifferentiating reduction of all tension, the self-destruction seen in an individual like Dylann Roof, and in Foucault's characterization of the Nazi state as absolutely racist, absolutely murderous, and absolutely suicidal.

In a summary statement, Charny writes:

> Genocidal evil is normal (common) in history and normal (readily available) in our human potential; but it is, by every sane standard, distinctly abnormal (undesirable). I think that seeing genocide as the ultimate expression of a disturbed balance between strength and weakness—an extreme

> form of pseudo strength that is as psychotic as the maddest form of mental weakness and incompetence—may open the door to a solution to the conceptual dilemma in psychology that we have not known how to call this very abnormal (evil) and antilife act what it really is: profoundly abnormal.
> (pp. 340–341)

To use words like "cancer" and "psychosis" suggests illnesses that have a life of their own, beyond conscious control. This might lead one to think that those who commit genocide or racist murder, when tried, could deserve an insanity defense. This was what Dylann Roof's lawyer attempted, and this was why Roof dismissed him. In a sense, Roof echoed Charny's position that we are "responsible for what we choose, knowingly or unknowingly" (p. 210). Of course, he took responsibility for his murders in a normally psychotic way. He was without guilt and maintained his belief in the necessity of race war. He said that he had planned to kill himself after his murders (rest, suicide). He then sought the death penalty. Is it possible to take responsibility for the cancer or psychosis of genocide? At the end of our last chapter, we asked an almost unthinkable question: to prevent genocide, must *Homo sapiens* take on responsibility for its own evolution? In *Why War* (to which we will return in our last chapter), Einstein asks, "Is it possible to control man's mental evolution so as to make him proof against the psychoses of hate and destructiveness?" (S.E. 22, p. 201). This impossible question is intrinsic to the genocide principle.

Note

1 If one looks at the life story of Dylann Roof, this describes him well.

7 Permanent Security

A. Dirk Moses' *The Problems of Genocide: Permanent Security and the Language of Transgression* challenges much of what we have seen so far. Moses states his position from the first page: "Genocide is a problem in two ways: not only the terrible fact of mass death, but also how the relatively new idea and law of genocide organizes and distorts our thinking about civilian (that is, noncombatant) destruction" (p. 1). He alleges that what gets distorted is the normative perspective on civilian immunity from attack. Why? Because when genocide becomes the "crime of crimes," one can be blinded to

> other types of humanly caused civilian death, like bombing cities and the 'collateral damage' of missile and drone strikes, blockades and sanctions. In other words, talk of genocide functions ideologically to detract attention from systematic violence perpetrated by governments, including Western ones [...] this violence is the consequence of 'permanent security' imperatives: the striving of States, and armed groups seeking to found states, to make themselves invulnerable to threats. Permanent security is the unobtainable goal of absolute safety that necessarily results in civilian casualties by its paranoid tendency to indiscriminate violence. To solve the problem of genocide concealing permanent security, this book proposes replacing the former with the latter: permanent security should be illegal.
>
> (p. 1)

If Moses is correct, then the concept of genocide might have done more harm than good. But is he correct? Or has he valuably discerned what one might call "*some* of the problems of genocide"? Can one expand the concept of genocide in conjunction with the problem of permanent security?

In order to answer these questions, I am choosing Moses' use of the word "paranoid" as a leitmotif. He uses it to characterize the "indiscriminate violence" of permanent security. It is a word we have encountered many times before. In the chapter on Kiernan we introduced Klein's idea of the paranoid-schizoid position to understand the unconscious dynamics of genocide; we

DOI: 10.4324/9781003562870-8

used the same concept in the chapters on Bauman, Foucault, Waller, and Weisband. We will see that Moses also uses (or at least alludes to), the same concept to explain permanent security. Could the way that his argument not only requires the use of the word "paranoid" but also leads to the paranoid-schizoid position be the bridge between genocide and permanent security?

Moses makes a compelling ethical argument:

> I dispute the 'doctrine of double effect' that permits the killing of innocents as a side-effect of a moral end, like self-defense. What does it matter to civilians if they are killed by violence inflicted with genocidal or military intent? And what if global policing is intrinsic to national security policy, thereby entailing constant military action—the 'infinity,' 'forever,' 'endless,' or 'permanent' wars in which some states are engaged?
>
> (p. 2)

Permanent war is another name for permanent security. Permanent security itself is self-defense and self-preservation. When Freud postulated a "purified pleasure ego" that creates a hated object, he then spoke about the self-preservative drive to destroy that object. This is the *paranoid* form of necessary self-defense.

In *Society Must be Defended,* Foucault extended the logic of this idea. Recall his theory of power as a theory of war. Power, even political power, is "war by other means." Political power then is on the side of "real battles, burning towns, ravaged fields, the innocent dead" (p. 50) and "elementary brutality" (p. 55). In a sense Foucault has anticipated Moses' argument. The "defense of society" (or search for "permanent security") is endless war, with the inevitable "innocent dead." In Moses' words: *"the continuous killing of civilians becomes the norm rather than confined to occasional wars"* (p. 3; author's emphasis), because people are considered combatants, not noncombatants: "...such practices are not so new: they are intrinsic to the global settler colonial expansion of Europe and its state model since the late fifteenth century" (pp. 3–4).

Aren't such practices much older than that? Moses himself speaks of "the violence of imperial expansion and consolidation that has marked human relations for millennia" (p. 11). The Athenian massacre of Melos occurred in the context of colonial expansion. The Biblical descriptions of the extermination of the Amalekites might be called a permanent security operation: wiping out the enemy who attacked you prevents reoccurrence. Whether indiscriminate violence against civilians dates to the late fifteenth century, or is much older, once "citizens are presumed guilty by association with enemy combatants ... we verge on the *mental world* of genocide: entire peoples as enemies whose members are collectively guilty, or at least expendable" (p. 4; my emphasis). There is, then, a "mental world of genocide" for Moses. It is intrinsic to "permanent security."

Again using the concept of "the mental world of genocide," Moses addresses the questions of race and identity. Genocide itself

> presumes the existence of identity-based groups as the building blocks of humanity that are targeted on the basis of this identity: by racial, ethnic, or religious hatred. In this categorization, populations comprise ethnic majorities and minorities as political facts. They are understood as political agents with ontological status rather than the outcomes of complex processes of racialization. This presupposition of fixed identities flies in the face of the fact that people have multiple, layered identities [...] When politics is imagined in sectarian terms, as ethnic struggle, *we* are inhabiting the *mental world of genocide* rather than thinking beyond it. Another problem of genocide, then, is its participation in the discursive construction of identity-based violence against civilians.
>
> (p. 12; my emphases)

Who is the "we" inhabiting the mental world of genocide? For perpetrators of genocide, certainly there are fixed racial identities. Such fixed racial identities have what Moses calls "political" and "ontological status." They concretely embody who is to be protected, who is the enemy, and within what boundaries. Is Moses' "we," then, anyone who imagines politics as "ethnic struggle"? At first it appears so, but then he says that the concept of genocide itself participates in the "construction of identity-based violence against civilians." In other words, "the mental world of genocide" is in the concept of genocide itself. Moses takes this as a problem, but is it? To understand genocide is precisely to understand why it is always a question of "racialization" *as politics*.

This too was Foucault's point about sovereignty, race, and war. Once the sovereign right to kill becomes a question of populations, the state itself creates a "superrace" and a "subrace." The "subrace is permanently, ceaselessly infiltrating the social body" (p. 61). Thus, the "appearance of a State racism: a racism that society will direct against itself, against its own elements and its own products. This is the internal racism of permanent purification" (pp. 61–62). Permanent purification: permanent security. And the idea that the state creates its racial–political enemy returns us to the logic of the purified pleasure ego and the paranoid-schizoid position. For both, the persecutory object is the projected version of the subject's self-destructiveness, which can then contaminate "us," calling for purification.

Moses proposes a sharp distinction between politically motivated racism and hatred. He is addressing another problem of genocide: the elimination of politically motivated mass murder from the Genocide Convention. Moses traces this back to Lemkin's list of national, ethnic, racial, and religious crimes against people, thereby "excluding other categories of civilians" (p. 17), most notably political groups. (The United States and the USSR opposed the original Genocide Convention; the United States, because its racial policies left it open to the charge of genocide, and the USSR because its politically motivated mass murders did the same.) Moses contends that the elimination of political groups from the "crime of crimes" allows nations to avoid the charge of genocide by claiming that it is acting for political reasons (p. 17). The "ethnic definition" of genocide, then, conceives it as "an irrational hate crime: innocent, blameless victims are attacked for racial rather than for political reasons ... Primordial antipathy or ideological racism, instead of rational political considerations, are supposed to motivate the perpetrator" (p. 18).

The problem with Moses' argument here is that it eliminates the "mental world of genocide" from its understanding of politics. Moses knows that he cannot eliminate racial hatred from politically motivated mass murder: "Security and racial animus intersect ... security and hatred accompany one another" (p. 19). What he seems not to appreciate is that when states claim to commit mass murder for security reasons, as is almost always the case, they also claim *not* to be motivated by hatred, but by the necessity to eliminate the contaminating enemy within. Again, paranoia: once an enemy has been created by projection, it is only reasonable to protect oneself against it. But everything hinges on this paranoid logic, as Moses knows.

Moses claims that the use of the atomic bomb against Hiroshima and Nagasaki is precisely the kind of security operation he has in mind: mass murder of civilians as combatants. This is a necessary point. But when he contends that the problem of genocide is that it does not understand genocide as a political crime in the name of permanent security, he does not grasp why, as he says, "security and hatred accompany one another." "Accompany" captures the essential: as soon as there is hatred, there is the necessity of security. And of impossible *permanent* security. Impossible because, whether in Freud's, Klein's, or Foucault's senses, the enemy will always be recreated; hence "permanent purification," permanent war. The "mental world of genocide" is one in which the impossibility of eliminating racial difference itself creates the normal psychosis of attempting to control the uncontrollable. Uncontrollable racial difference then becomes fixed, political, "ontological" identity, as Moses contends.

He comes up against this issue when he says that:

> Permanent security implicates racialization when it is combined with securitization: identifying a group as threatening. Persecution does not occur without securitization even if victims experience their persecution as the outcome of hatred, because this is the emotion they *discern* in the perpetrators. The social fact of racial or religious difference or even prejudice does not cause genocidal violence, however [...] permanent security is an impossible and immoral aspiration that drives states and para-states to kill innocent people in the name of ending vulnerability by imposing their regime—forever.
>
> (p. 42; my emphasis)

When Moses says that racial or religious difference does not cause genocidal violence he simply does not take into account the narcissistically violent response to difference, another aspect of "the mental world of genocide." Narcissistic in that it is both self-preservative and self-destructive, as we have seen throughout. Moses acknowledges that victims "discern" hatred in the perpetrators. "Discern" seems to imply seeing beyond the obvious. That is, even if the perpetrators seem to act out of reasonable necessity, the victims "discern" that they are acting out of hatred. Are the victims wrong? And when Moses says that permanent security is an "impossible and immoral aspiration" that kills innocent people "in the name of ending vulnerability … forever," he is again correct. Kiernan spelled out the "forever," utopian vision of genocide.

Moses' use of the term "permanent security" is deliberately provocative. He has taken it from Otto Ohlendorf, a Nazi commander in Eastern Europe who oversaw the mass murder of Jews (p. 34). At his trial in 1947, Ohlendorf did not typically "cite superior orders" (p. 35) to defend himself. Rather he claimed that his actions were necessary to achieve "permanent security" (p. 35). Moses cites a speech of Hitler's in 1939 that speaks of the "feeling of security" to be achieved by the ethnic reordering of the continent, including "the attempt to order and regulate the Jewish problem" (p. 35). Moses says that this implies a "radically new temporal structure," the elimination of not only "immediate threats, but future threats" (p. 35). (Again, Kiernan makes this point.) Consistently, Moses understands this new temporal structure in relation to paranoia. The attempt to "close the gap between *perceived* insecurity and permanent security" (p. 35; my emphasis) "…entails a fatally restless and dynamic process indentured to a paranoid subject who not only perceives grave threats but *manufactures* circumstances in which they become self fulfilling prophecies" (p. 35; my emphasis). Moses contends that Ohlendorf gave a "devastatingly clear" account of Nazi motivations that applies to all instances of civilian deaths in the name of permanent security. He says that we would prefer to "ignore" this account because of its "provenance" (p. 35). The paranoid subject always manufactures the threats that compel self-defense. But why doesn't Moses understand that this process would not exist without the projection of self-destructiveness, and the consequent hatred? Does he take Ohlendorf at face value, not looking at why "extermination policies made perfect sense to its followers" (p. 36)? In other words, that extermination policies aiming at permanent security reflect the paranoid mental world of genocide?

Moses' ethical position valuably forces one to look at the continuum between what he calls "liberal permanent security" (e.g., Western nations' colonizing wars in the putative name of spreading civilization) and "illiberal permanent security" (e.g., Nazi wars in the name of a "thousand year Reich"). Analogously, he is asking us to see that, for the civilian dead, there is no difference between war crimes, crimes against humanity, and genocide. He is clear that the link between racialization and permanent security reflects the "mental world of genocide." His protest against the exclusion of political groups from the Genocide Convention is not unique. But his contention that what we now call genocide *must* be considered a political crime committed to achieve permanent security artificially separates politics from hatred, taking perpetrators' contentions that they are not acting out of hate at face value. Again, it is as if the "mental world of genocide" is not created by unconscious processes.

Some crucial passages illustrate this problem. Moses contends that permanent security is governed "more by fantastical security imperatives—paranoid threat assessments—than by the aesthetic of racial purity as implied by the Holocaust" (p. 273). "Paranoid threat assessments" are precisely those in which the enemy has been created by projection. The threat is indeed "fantastical." As Moses knows, such a fantastically created enemy is endlessly recreated, which is why permanent security is permanent purification. And as he also knows, "racialization" reflects "the mental world of genocide." "Racialization" itself is the process in which racial difference becomes fixed identity, the fixed identity of the always recreated enemy and, thus, the narcissistic violence of "fantastical security imperatives." If all of this is the case, then hatred *is* politics; hatred and politics are joined in the unconscious process which makes politics *appear* to be governed by rational considerations, once the "fantastical" is taken as the real. This is why the victims "discern" hatred in perpetrators, no matter the appearances.

Moses continues:

> the conventional view suggests a hierarchy between types of human destruction. Nonpolitical violence is considered worse because it targets innocent victims of paranoid and ultimately inexplicable racial hysteria, while political violence is an explicable outcome of interethnic conflict [...] . This distinction between political nongenocide on the one hand, and racial, ideological genocide on the other, conceals the combatant/civilian distinction *within* such groups. It ignores the fact that both categories of violence contain massacres of civilians who pose no objective threat to perpetrators.
>
> (pp. 273–274; author's emphasis)

When Moses refers to "inexplicable racial hysteria" one can recall the passage from *Groups Psychology* in which Freud spoke of the primal hatred of racial difference that he could not explain; perhaps Moses means something akin to what Freud meant. For the observer such racial "hysteria" is indeed baffling, especially because it makes a nonthreatening group into an existential menace. Moses' point that the "combatant/civilian distinction" is concealed in both "political nongenocide" and "racial, ideological genocide" is unclear. In the Holocaust, were Jews combatants? Only in Himmler's sense as "this people who want to destroy us." One might contend that in Rwanda the historical antagonism between Tutsis and Hutus might justify seeing the Tutsis as combatants, but can one say the same for the allegedly "Tutsified"

Hutus who were slaughtered, or the allegedly "Vietnamized" Cambodians who too were slaughtered? Moses does want to make the point that there are mass deaths of both civilians and combatants, and there he is obviously correct. In effect, he demonstrates that the "mental world of genocide" is at work in both instances.

Moses offers a further analysis of the paranoid mental world of genocide:

> The paranoia often emanates from traumatic and humiliating experiences of loss and occupation [...] the nature of traumatized consciousness means that past events are never really past: the past can repeat itself [...] There are no limits in dealing with traitors in emergency circumstances. This dynamic indicates that [the] distinction between violence based on (nonpolitical) hallucinatory threat perceptions and (political) real conflict is misleading. In fact, permanent security crimes are based on traumatic memories of past events in which 'disloyal' peoples [...] are held collectively guilty and then collectively deported or destroyed preemptively to prevent the feared repetition of traumatic experiences. For the paranoid subject, the hallucinatory is all too real. Paradoxically, then, the policy prescriptions that follow from paranoid threat assessments seem all-too-rational.
>
> (p. 274)

Weisband has a similar analysis:

> perpetrators [...] revel in their absolute power, but simultaneously [...] project hatred, revenge, and revulsion onto their victims, who are reified and thus made to appear, at first in fantasy but eventually in ideological constructions, as the very incarnation of the shame, humiliation, and loss against which the perpetrators also seek to defend.
>
> (p. 10)

Whether in Moses or Weisband, the point is that when perpetrators repeat trauma, shame, and humiliation by projecting them *into* (Klein) others, the "hallucinatory" or the fantastical *is* the real. Apparently, rational, *political* security concerns express this process. This is why Ohlendorf's claim to have acted in the name of permanent security was *in fact* intrinsic to a genocidal project motivated by hatred *as* politics. When Moses continues the analysis that tries to eliminate hatred from politics, he says that mass violence against civilians is justified by "frightened patriots and those indoctrinated in paranoia. That does not mean they do not hate the group they attacked; they do, often driven by revenge ... It means that fear and paranoia rather than antipathy inaugurate the campaigns" (p. 275). What is the difference between "fear and paranoia" and "antipathy"? That the "distinction between violence based on (nonpolitical) hallucinatory threat perceptions and (political) real conflict is misleading" again demonstrates how "the mental world of genocide" is operative in both cases.

Speaking of the Armenian genocide, Moses says that the Young Turks were determined to prevent an Armenian state. Their aim was to reduce the Armenian population, which could only be done "in a genocidal way" (p. 275). What he calls the "disturbing lesson" is "the relation of *raison d'etat* and criminality" (p. 275). His conclusion is that:

> wicked, crazed, racist, and authoritarian leaders are unnecessary for the criminality of permanent security [...] The fatal logic of permanent security is the paranoid ascription of collective guilt and then preemptive action [...] In this sense, racial fantasies and security paranoia intersect with fatal consequences for victim groups.
>
> (p. 275)

Again, whether liberal or illiberal in Moses' terms, killing civilians in the name of permanent security participates in the "mental world of genocide." The concept of "permanent security" is an essential *aspect* of understanding genocide itself.

In *Group Psychology and the Analysis of the Ego* Freud alleged that groups are held together by identification with a leader. Integrating Klein into this understanding, we have alleged that participation in genocide depends upon identification with a leader who embodies the paranoid-schizoid position. When Moses says that "wicked, crazed, racist, and authoritarian leaders are unnecessary for the criminality of permanent security," he might be making an argument that is sometimes valid. But his own logic explains such criminality in terms of paranoia. And even the paranoid-schizoid position.

> Political paranoia is a form of projective identification in which the subject displaces intolerable, negative feelings onto others who thence incarnate the disavowed, persecutory self. By externalizing internally experienced feelings of worthlessness, they are rendered manageable, and positive self image is maintained—though at considerable cost: the construction of a delusional reality. The subject is always the victim and the other the persecutor. Political paranoia is at once a psychological regression to a child-like 'paranoid-schizoid position' and an interpretive disorder constituted by hysterical threat assessments.
>
> (p. 322)

Moses here does not directly cite Klein, but others who have used her work (including Semelin, Chapter 8). He has given a good capsule summary. He understands that projective identification creates a persecutory enemy, such that a positive (idealized) self-image is maintained, at the cost of constructing a delusional reality. These enemies become the victims who "represent"—or delusionally *are*—the "abject attributes" of the "paranoid persecutor" (p. 322; see Weisband). Hence, any empathy for the victims is a threat: "to imaginatively occupy their subject position would entail interjecting [sic, but he clearly means "introjecting"] the intolerable feelings that were split off in the first place" (p. 322). This is a fine understanding of Klein's idea that depressive position responsibility for the "disaster created by one's own sadism" creates intolerable anxiety, and reinforcement of paranoid-schizoid mechanisms. These mechanisms then become the political, whether there is a leader who promotes them or they are collectively accepted (Foucault's "state racism").

Moses, then, does understand the paranoid-schizoid mechanisms that create the political. In his terms these mechanisms produce the imperative for *permanent*, "forever," security, the fantasy of omnipotent control. Such omnipotent control is intrinsic to the idea of sovereignty. The sovereign state's freedom to kill, whether its own people, or others, is the *conjoint* problem of genocide and permanent security. At times, Moses does put it this way. Addressing the purported distinction between mass murder of civilians that would end after a war (e.g., the fire bombing of Dresden) and the mass murder of a target group (e.g., the Jews) that would have continued should a perpetrator country (e.g., Germany) win a war, Moses says that

> killing hundreds of thousands of civilians was legitimate in the course of military operations, but not to avert a future threat. The Allies and Nazis were operating with different conceptions of warfare. This was one difference between liberal and illiberal permanent security.
>
> (p. 237)

He then asks:

> what if military necessity and genocide had been joined [...]? What if the recourse to military necessity in which civilians are murdered [...] were considered genocide as well, because it was driven not by racial hatred but by the quest for what Ohlendorf called permanent security? Why is murder on apparent racial grounds the 'worst of all possible motives'?
>
> (p. 237)

The great difficulty here is that the exercise of state sovereignty, whether liberal or illiberal, indeed can conjoin permanent security and genocide almost interchangeably; this is why Moses can say that "military necessity" can be genocidal. But the question he elides is precisely the question of sovereignty. To make permanent security illegal, is essentially to make sovereignty illegal. When international law attempts to make "murder on apparent racial grounds" illegal, it too elides the question of sovereignty. Or rather, confronts it *and* elides it.

Moses could disagree with my contention that he elides the question of sovereignty, because he does take it up, providing some essential historical material. After the Armenian genocide, Vespasian Pella in *La criminalité collective des états et le droit pénal de l'avenir* (*The Collective Criminality of States and the Penal Law of the Future*, 1925) wrote of "crimes so grave as to justify violating the principle of state sovereignty in the interests of 'restoring the moral order which must reign in the whole of humanity' " (cited by Moses, p. 153). Andre Mandelstam in *Le sort de l'empire Ottoman* (*The Fate of the Ottoman Empire*, 1917) rejected the theory that "rights inhered in the state," instead proclaiming the "sovereignty of law above the state" (cited by Moses, p. 155). Later, Mandelstam advocated an "international regime of protection; rather than some states' sovereignty being porous every states' should be, even if a little" (p. 155).

All of this suggests what became the UN's adoption of the doctrine of Responsibility to Protect. In 1999, Kofi Annan, then Secretary-General of the UN, which under his leadership had done nothing to intervene in the Rwandan genocide and "ethnic cleansing" in Bosnia, proposed changing the definition of state sovereignty. Basically, Annan was saying that the state is the servant of its people, not vice versa. His idea was that traditional notions of state sovereignty cannot do justice to individual aspirations to fundamental freedoms. Two years later the International Commission on Intervention and State Sovereignty went further, stating that "defense of state sovereignty … does not include any claim of the unlimited power of a state to do what it wants to its own people" (p. 8). Sovereignty implies dual responsibility: to respect the sovereignty of other states and to respect the basic rights of all people in the state (p. 8). This maintenance of state sovereignty changes sovereignty as control to sovereignty as responsibility. In 2005 the doctrine of sovereignty as responsibility was adopted by the General Assembly. (Moses briefly refers to this p. 50.) A 2019 UN report on what came to be called Responsibility to Protect bleakly stated that everything was "moving in the wrong direction."

In one sense, Moses has anticipated the inevitable problem of this attempt to address the right to kill (Foucault) built into the notion of sovereignty. As he has said, perpetrators' empathy with victims of genocide/permanent security is impossible, because it would entail "interjecting" (introjecting) everything that has been projected onto (into) them. As per Klein, there is no depressive position without a paranoid-schizoid position. This is what the earlier proposals to limit state sovereignty in the wake of the Armenian genocide, and the more current one in Responsibility to Protect, do not take into account. It is why Moses wants to make permanent security illegal. His entire analysis links permanent security to the paranoid-schizoid position. What I have called his eliding of the question of sovereignty, then, is not the recognition of the problem of sovereignty, already understood after World War I. It is the question of understanding that whether one is speaking of genocide and/or permanent security, there is no possibility of making the paranoid-schizoid position illegal. This is why such a well-intended idea as Responsibility to Protect—in effect, making the depressive position the definition of sovereignty—has failed. Moses elides this issue when he says that "Although the current 'responsibility to protect' eschews the language of imperial humanitarian interventionism, its declarations about competent governance ... embody familiar colonial assumptions about Western pre-eminence while screening out the dependence of Western state-building on imperial domination" (p. 500). The point is well taken, but does not deal with the way that the paranoid mental world of genocide is built into sovereignty, i.e., permanent security. When Moses says that "Mass crimes are thus seen as extreme and rare irruptions of violence into an otherwise healthy normality rather than as the manifestations of potentials immanent in hierarchical and exploitative relationships" (p. 479), he is recognizing that the violence of hierarchy and exploitation—sovereignty—is irreducible.

When we think of sovereign states, we usually imagine states within defined borders. However, sovereignty almost always implies ethnic uniformity—a racial boundary. "Liberal permanent security" will have it that ethnic "others" are to be tolerated. Moses contends that

> talk of toleration is a logical corollary of the ethnically defined nation-state that constitutes the geopolitical imaginary of the UN: each 'people' housed in 'its' state. The genocide discourse does not challenge this ethnic construction of the state and its divine cartography: the assumption that a *Volk* governs and reproduces itself through the state and that others are to be tolerated. These assumptions presuppose that outsiders remain outsiders, foreign bodies in the body politic to be at best tolerated and, if they seem to develop their own collective will and are perceived as threatening, to be suppressed, expelled or destroyed.
>
> (p. 494)

In other words, "genocide discourse" potentially participates in the reasoning that makes mass crimes possible. The deliberate use of the word "*Volk*," with its Nazi connotations, suggests that to consider the Holocaust a "hate crime"—the Jews as "foreign bodies" in an Aryan nation—problematically supports the "geopolitical imaginary" of "each 'people' housed in 'its' state."

There is a compelling logic here: Moses is saying that to believe in the ethnic uniformity of the sovereign state contains the seeds of violence. However, if one understands that the dynamics of the "mental world of genocide" are at play here, there are more ways to conceptualize why this "geopolitical imaginary" is both geographical and ethnic. Above, we saw Kiernan speak of the "dominating ambition" in genocide as a "phobia of contamination." We extended this point by taking "phobia" in the psychoanalytic sense: what one is apparently afraid of is not what one is unconsciously afraid of. The "phobia of contamination" expresses the fear that "they" are already inside us. "We" are porous. The insistence on intact geographic–ethnic boundaries, then, is a projective defense against what is intolerably "inside," and what has the insidious capacity to get inside no matter how strong the boundary, precisely because the boundary will always be porous. Hence, the "Jewish virus" to be eliminated in the Thousand Year Reich—or the Tutsified Hutus, or the Vietnamized Cambodians. Permanent security as permanent purification.

Bauman too analyzed this issue: "The objects of antisemitism occupy as a rule the semantically confusing and psychologically unnerving status of foreigners inside, thereby striding a vital boundary which ought to be clearly drawn and kept intact and impregnable" (p. 34). Waller similarly said that when "group membership is seen as impermeable and fixed, the potential to view other groups as *perpetual* threats is heightened" (p. 174; my emphasis). The quest for permanent security/purification is the unconscious attempt to make the porous impermeable. The "mental world of genocide" translated into geography. And which geographical boundary has ever been completely impermeable? When have there ever not been "foreigners inside"?

Let us return to our point of departure, and Moses' conclusion:

> The hope of this book is to promote civilian protection by a revaluation of international law [...] That would entail making permanent security a crime to discourage states from exceeding legitimate security concerns: so they do not engage in civilian destruction, try to impose ethnic or religious homogeneity on diverse populations, or attempt to dominate regions, indeed the world, with the attendant extreme violence.
>
> (p. 511)

I do not dispute the existence of "legitimate security concerns" (Ukraine today, Poland and Czechoslovakia at the beginning of WW II, among thousands of transhistorical examples). But how to adjudicate "legitimate security concerns" once a politics of hate *creates* the dangerous "foreigners within"? Perhaps Moses' references to paranoia and the paranoid-schizoid position point the way to an answer. Is it outlandish to think that a global recognition of these unconscious dynamics is possible? That there could be a psychoanalytically informed way to address why this danger will always be present if there have to be sovereign states? Of course, psychoanalysis itself would predict why there would have to be enormous resistance to such thinking. But addressing that resistance would at least entail an objective assessment of what is at stake.

8 Purification and Destruction

In *Purify and Destroy* French sociologist Jacques Semelin offers his explanation of genocide. His title once more recalls Freud on the purified pleasure ego: in the name of self-preservation, the ego hates and attempts of *destroy* the object onto whom its own internal tensions have been projected, hence *purifying* itself. Semelin does not refer to this theory. However, the consonance of his title with Freud makes vivid that rigorous thought about genocide must be psychoanalytic. Semelin does recognize this point. Let us follow him up to its assertion.

He begins with the common question of how "ordinary people" can commit such acts. The very "incoherence" of this reality makes understanding perpetrators a "moral obligation" (pp. 2–3). While starting from his sociological perspective, Semelin says that research from "all branches of the social sciences is necessary" (pp. 2–3). He puts genocide under the general rubric of "massacre," which he defines as "a *form of action that is most often collective and aimed at destroying non-combatants*" (p. 4; author's emphasis). (He later makes the point that "massacre" originally meant putting an animal to death, e.g., during a hunt. He relates this etymology to the "bestialization," the de-humanizing of victims of genocide [p. 38].) "Massacre" takes him to Foucault. The focus is on the power to destroy (man or beast one might say), and as *per* Foucault "the body is the privileged receptacle of power's will" (cited, p. 5). Hence, states can set in motion political practices of purification and destruction of the "social body" (p. 6; e.g., necessary action against the "Jewish virus").

Because mass murder is "absolutely mind-boggling," Semelin says, one might be "paralyzed by his subject matter" (p. 6). This could lead to the "cliche of conventional discourse" that genocide is "unthinkable" (p. 7). To counter the cliché he says that "Of course genocide is thinkable—unfortunately it is too thinkable" (p. 7). Nonetheless, "the closer one draws to the fundamental core of human cruelty, the more he is faced with a sort of 'black hole' that resists any sort of understanding via the intellect" (p. 7). But the "black holes" that resist understanding by ordinary intellect are precisely the province of psychoanalysis, as Semelin will acknowledge.

DOI: 10.4324/9781003562870-9

Even before this acknowledgment, Semelin recognizes that genocide is a question of mind. (Recall Moses on "the mental world of genocide.") Massacres:

> are mainly born out of a mental process, a way of seeing some 'Other' being, of stigmatizing him, debasing him, and obliterating him before actually killing him. This is always a complex mental process, and it usually takes time to mature. But it can also develop at astounding speed.
>
> (p. 9)

Semelin is clear about the paradox of boundaries: the debased enemy who supposedly comes from "outside our borders" is "also within them" (p. 9). (Recall Bauman on the "viscous," boundary-blurring conceptual Jew.) And as per Freud in *Group Psychology* ... Semelin sees the essential role of the leader. While there may have been "pre-existing antipathies" between groups, they "...only really gain in magnitude if leaders organize them ... The leader affirms what is happening, why it is happening, and who is responsible" (p. 13).

The leader affirms, explains, and blames. This allows him to assert a crisis: "our" identity is threatened. To deal with this "imaginary" destabilization of identity, the leader responds with "... an imaginary construct that restructures the crisis on a new foundation. The collective anxiety of the population is transformed into an intense fear of a highly dangerous enemy, a 'cancer'" (p. 16). (Charny called genocide "the human cancer," perhaps because of the universality of the "imaginary construct" that the bestial threatening other is also a disease.) The "treatment" of this cancer can only be the destruction of its agents. This produces "a fantasy of all-powerfulness in which this 'us' is regenerated by destroying 'them'" (p. 17), thereby ensuring "the omnipotence of us" (p. 17). Semelin calls this the "inextricable link between the *imaginaire* of death and the *imaginaire* of omnipotence" (p. 17). This "inextricable link" is an "archaic structure" that affects "the very foundations of the human psyche as explained, for example, by psychoanalysis" (p. 17).

What psychoanalytic explanation of the archaic link between the *imaginaire* of death and the *imaginaire* of omnipotence does Semelin choose? He briefly refers to Freud's contribution to the dialogue with Einstein in *Why War?* There Freud spoke about the death drive, the human capacity for self-destruction. Semelin calls this a "pseudo-explanation"; man tends to destroy himself because there is a destructive drive (p. 18). However, he thinks that Klein "went further" and gives the familiar description of the paranoid-schizoid and depressive positions. His dismissal of the death drive, however, obscures the fundamental role that *projection* of it plays in Klein's work. This explains why the perceived enemy is a version of oneself, akin to the purified pleasure ego. Nonetheless, referencing Italian analyst Franco Fornari's analysis of *Why War?,* he credits Fornari for giving the same importance to the depressive position as Klein—"saving the love object through which he feels alive to the extent of sacrificing himself out of love for this object" (p. 19). (It is unclear why Semelin speaks of self-sacrifice, rather than *responsibility* for one's aggression, as does Klein, unless he equates the two.) The essential point is that agreeing with Klein and Fornari, Semelin sees the depressive position as "the origin of civilization" (p. 19).

Starting with *Totem and Taboo* and culminating in *Civilization and Its Discontents,* Freud had put the prohibition of murder in this originating position. But what is prohibited is always *there,* which then actually puts murder in the originating position. Semelin thinks that Freud's attribution of guilt over the murder of the primal father, and subsequent establishment of laws against murder, can "inhibit individual violence but not war" (p. 19). This is too simple for at least two reasons. First, once murder is in the originating position, the law that prohibits murder can also prescribe murder, whether in the form of the death penalty, or even lawful obedience to the sovereign god's or state's command to kill. Second, is Freud's point in *Thoughts for the Times on War and Death* that the state prohibits violence in order to monopolize it. One can ascribe this monopolization to Foucault's definition of sovereignty: the right to kill. The sovereign right to kill is the omnipotence Semelin himself links to "the *imaginaire* of death."

Like Foucault, Semelin says that politics is a means of pursuing war, and he adds as a means of pursuing war against civilians (p. 329). This was Moses' topic—destruction of civilians in the name of permanent security. Moses referenced the paranoid-schizoid position, which we had already integrated with Foucault's analysis of war and state racism. Similarly, Semelin, citing Fornari, says that war is "the epitome of the paranoid-schizoid position: one survives by killing the enemy" (p. 20), a "psychotic illusion" (p. 20). Semelin explains this via Rene Spitz on stranger anxiety, the stage at which the typical eight-month-old baby attributes aggressive intent to an unknown, *unfamiliar* person, without that person's having manifested any hostility (p. 20). Fornari, extending this idea, says that "societies, with respect to war, are conditioned from a psychological standpoint to situate themselves at the level of anxiety of an eight month old child" (cited, p. 20). (Recall Charny's statement that the correspondence between the paranoid-schizoid position and the relations between states is "impressive.") Stranger anxiety is universal. However, as Semelin says, the "psychotic illusion" that one survives by *killing* the enemy is greater than stranger anxiety. The unquestioned belief in such an illusion, in which "the imaginary and the real" are conflated, is explained by Bion's idea of projective identification against one's own mind: one's paranoid-schizoid conflicts are lodged within the other, who then is a crazed threat to oneself.

This is the mechanism that the leader depends upon, whether consciously or not. The leader can affirm, explain, and blame *effectively* because he idealizes this mechanism. As Semelin stresses, he promises omnipotence, and intuitively "knows" that the paranoid-schizoid mechanisms in everyone *need* this promise in order to fight for self-preservation. In other words, the group *needs* the leader's narcissism. The mutual reinforcing of projection of the death drive, of splitting into idealized good and persecutory bad objects, of projective identification against one's own mind, are all operative in the leader's narcissistic grandiosity. This is why we have spoken of the leader as an idealized pseudo-good object. "Pseudo-good" because the promise of *omnipotent* destruction of the "persecutor" is self-destructive. And this idealized, self-destructive self-preservation frequently becomes morality itself. "Anchoring mass murder on the side of morality gives it an extraordinarily destructive force, and over a long period of time" (p. 255).

Thus, perpetrators believe that they are on a moral crusade to save civilization, while the observer sees them as barbaric. We come back to the question of the origin, the possibility of civilization—the prohibition of murder or the depressive position? Semelin had objected to Freud on the grounds that guilt over murder could prevent individual violence, but not war. However, one could say the same about the depressive position. Responsibility for one's aggression prevents individual acts of sadism and destruction. How to put the depressive position at the origin of group existence, of civilization itself? And how to keep in mind Freud's idea about the state's monopolization of violence?

Semelin seems not to attend to Klein's idea that achievement of the depressive position is tenuous and anxiety-laden. She says that the necessary integration of good and bad creates extreme anxiety over loss of the good. Certainly, this applies to the relation of the group to the genocidal leader. To begin to see the cruelty and madness that the genocidal leader says is necessary for survival would be to lose the idealized, "good" leader. But this loss of the idealized object is also loss of the leader's promise of omnipotence. Without omnipotence one is subject to fear of chaotic loss of control, and even annihilation as per Bion. Klein did not include this idea in her conception of depressive anxiety. But it is why the state's *lawful* monopolization of violence, of the right to kill, is crucial. It builds paranoid-schizoid omnipotence into sovereignty. For the depressive position to be the origin of civilization—and not only acts of individual violence—states themselves would have to achieve the depressive position. Above, in Moses, we argued that this is the essence of Responsibility to Protect. States would have to become *responsible* for their violence against their own citizens (genocide) and against other states. This entails tolerating the anxieties related to loss of omnipotence, of sovereignty—which is why Responsibility to Protect has failed. If civilization assumes any form of sovereignty, whether religious or political, paranoid-schizoid mechanisms are inevitable.

Sovereignty also implies identity: we are citizens of a sovereign state; we are members of a religious group obedient to a sovereign god; we are by members of a superior ethnic group. Semelin does mention Freud on the narcissism of (minor) differences, although critically. He says that Freud does not take context sufficiently into account, i.e., does not describe the specific perception of difference that a group needs to buttress a sense of identity. Did Semelin read the passage in *Group Psychology* in which Freud spoke of a primally destructive response to racial or national difference? It seems not, but he accounts for identity formation in a way entirely applicable to that passage: "...identity is conceived through the perception of difference, giving substance both to the one and the Other ... this identity 'open' to another can retreat and withdraw into itself by establishing a criterion of exclusion from this Other" (p. 27). "Open" is a critical word here. It says that any sense of identity irreducibly comes from a relation to another. In principle, identity includes difference; there would be no identity if everyone were identical. Why, then, does it "withdraw into itself" *excluding* what it had to *include*? Why, in Semelin's resonant phrase, does identity become "the rage of Oneness" (p. 33)?

Here, one must return to Freud on life and death. The life drive, Eros, increases tension in the psyche by introducing fresh, *vital*, differences. But precisely because it is tension raising ("destabilizing" in Charny's expression), it is opposed by its counterpart, the tension reducing, dedifferentiating ("stabilizing") death drive. This is why Freud calls the life drive a "mischief maker" and spoke of the struggle against Eros. However, he did not apply this thinking to the primally destructive response to racial and national difference. Nor did he provide the basic analysis of identity and difference that Semelin provides here. Bauman had spoken of "adiaphoristic action," the downplaying of unpredictable, "*differentiating*, and thus potentially *divisive*, features" (p. 213; my emphases). Weisband said that "The unpredictable and the inconstant, the creative and the 'spontaneous surprise' in human exchange must be brought under *control* since they become anathema to sadistic aims that detest all forms of singularity and autonomy, *difference and otherness*" (p. 206; my emphases).

The leader "knows," i.e., intuitively feels, all of this. Because difference both constitutes and threatens identity it must be destroyed. The death drive is brought into operation against it. Thus, the greater the leaders' narcissistic promise of paranoid-schizoid omnipotence, the more he unites the group around exclusion of difference. This expands Freud's conception of how mutual identification with the leader holds the group together. Semelin cites Bartov, who said that the more Jews were dehumanized the more Hitler was deified (cited, p. 256), a precise description of these paranoid-schizoid mechanisms. The open relation to the different other is now *apparently* closed around an essentialized identity. Protection of this identity justifies continual killing, which can produce a feeling of immortality, omnipotence. But—and this is the "catch"—the originally included can never be permanently excluded. The enemy is always within, a beast, a disease. Hence the escalating dependence on the leader's imaginary omnipotence. Semelin's "rage of" (psychotic) purification by destruction.

The rage of oneness, purification by destruction, is paranoia: "...the word fits perfectly, since the structuring of these imaginary representations of the enemy is reminiscent of the descriptions psychiatry ascribes to paranoid personalities" (p. 44). Semelin calls it "delusional rationality" (p. 45), another way of thinking "normal psychosis," the usurpation of secondary process by primary process, or in Semelin's words "the permeability between the imaginary and the real" (p. 46). Semelin thinks that the paranoid discourse offered to the public is even more important than the leader. But even without a singular leader in genocide, the diffusion of this discourse by media takes on the leader's role; the media affirm, explain, and blame. This was spectacularly true of the use of the radio in Rwanda, where "accusation in the mirror" was a deliberate technique. Semelin also says that paranoid discourse creates a "security dilemma" (Moses), which makes "us" innocent of the "crime we will be accused of" because obviously we have to protect ourselves from "them," the ones who want to destroy "us." Destroy us, we might add, with their uncontrollable, divisive difference.

To exercise omnipotent control over uncontrollable difference, there must be a "symbolic barrier ... that cannot be crossed" (p. 49) between the included and the excluded. (Recall the role of mountains in Diamond's description of the hatreds between indigenous New Guineans.) This is the only way to establish security (Moses again). Semelin summarizes:

> this elemental psychological core, rooted in the *imaginaire* of early childhood, is at the basis of a process of violence that can lead to a massacre. We can suppose that this psychological core, precisely because it is elementary, is universal in human nature. A common denominator of the human species it transcends cultural differences. Of course its political realization varies from one country or continent to another: processes of violence will always vary in intensity and have individual characteristics.
>
> (p. 50)

Once this universal psychological core transcends cultural differences, it is at the origin of culture. In *Civilization and Its Discontents* Freud addressed primal violence, the foundational prohibition of it, and its inevitable resurfacing: "In consequence of this primary mutual hostility of human beings, civilized society is perpetually threatened with disintegration" (S.E. 21, p. 112). Further, this "inborn human inclination to 'badness', to aggressiveness and destructiveness," predisposes "to cruelty as well" (S.E. 21, p. 120). In a similar vein, Semelin writes:

> culture does not in itself have the faculty to lead man to free himself from violence. It is rather the contrary, that culture can supply him with the means to be more intelligent in exercising violence, and in resorting to cruelty.
>
> (p. 61)

As Semelin says, and Freud would agree, culture itself instrumentalizes violence and cruelty. In other words, culture cannot free man from violence because of the paranoid-schizoid mechanisms at its core. Culture in general, like the sovereign monopolization of violence in general, is *inimical* to the depressive position. But Semelin has alleged that the depressive position is the origin of civilization. Is it? Or is this not rather what one hopes eventually to be the case?

For it to be the case, civilization/culture would have to undergo the difficult journey through depressive anxiety. Once again we encounter the knot of sovereignty. "According to the principle of the sovereign territorial state arising from the 1648 treaty of Westphalia, the state can do whatever it deemed right within its borders" (p. 108). Hence, the familiar paradox: respect of sovereignty countenances genocide.[1] Semelin adduces the "experts" who "make the case for the principle of sovereignty being regulated, but not abandoned," while others "prefer to speak of 'responsibility to protect' (p. 110). Is there "a right and even a duty to intervene" or would this permit "intervention into former colonies"? (p. 110). Semelin skirts this knot when he says that it "is not the principle of sovereignty that causes violence, but the way states use it" (p. 109). If sovereignty is the right to kill, then violence is as much at its core as Semelin's elemental psychological core. Perhaps contradicting his thought that sovereignty does not cause violence, Semelin later writes: "...inventing the 'right to intervene' amounts to seeking to impose on governments a responsibility to protect that goes against their 'political nature' " (p. 163). Putting "right to intervene" and "political nature" between ironic scare quotes, while not similarly inflecting "responsibility to protect," illustrates the problem in the writing itself. Responsibility is not a right; political nature is actually the nature of elemental processes.

The inevitable, simple conclusion is that "...the practice of massacre would in reality be the sign not of a strong power but rather of a power that feels itself to be vulnerable, and which aspires, via massacre, to cease to be so" (p. 225). To be in the grips of this process is a political psychosis, driven to self-protective self-destruction. This is why Semelin makes the valid, but seemingly self-contradictory point, that one cannot apply the concept of intent to a power structure. This would be, he says, to "psychologize" it (pp. 178–179). What he means is that one cannot understand massacre in terms of a direct sequence of having the idea of destroying a group, planning the destruction, and then implementing it (pp. 178–179). Rather, one must attend to the "complexity of the development of such phenomena" (pp. 178–179). In other words, one has to understand the interaction of the elemental psychic forces in their specific context. But the overall point is that this then becomes a process with its own power, a process that those who believe they are justifiably asserting their *sovereign right to control what they cannot control*. Semelin cites a witness to the Rwandan genocide: it was "'a madness that went on all by itself'..." (p. 289). Charny: the cancer that cannot be stopped. This is the genocide principle in action.

Semelin provides a vivid description of the workings of the self-destructive, self-preservative genocide principle. The organization of the population to participate in massacre ends up:

> sucking the lifeblood out of the state like a vampire, so it becomes murderous of its own population or other populations falling under its control [...] This vampiric hold on power gives rise, in the state apparatus itself or in its orbit, to a new 'creature' conceived especially to dole out death.
>
> (p. 184)

(Kiernan and Foucault make the same point that genocide actually increases the vulnerability of the state, even exposing it to destruction.) Integrating the political analysis with the psychoanalytic perspective to explain the vampiric automaticity of the genocide principle, Semelin writes: "...power draws on identity, war on security, ideology on purity" (p. 229). And if this process of destruction is accepted collectively, it is precisely because it is "... '*grafted*' on to and feeds on, this imaginary base that every individual aspires to. It can therefore assume the dimensions of a full blown social incandescence—that of a purifying wave of destruction" (p. 229; author's emphasis).

This universal imaginary base is what Semelin has called the "black hole" of "the fundamental core of human cruelty" (p. 7). Is cruelty synonymous with sadism? This is another knot. On one hand, there is the common observation that most perpetrators were not manifestly sadistic. On the other, their manifest cruelty. Commenting on *Eichmann in Jerusalem,* and agreeing with Arendt on Eichmann's "terrifying inability to think," Semelin nevertheless says that Arendt does not tackle "the most enigmatic and uncomfortable dimension of all: that of cruelty, often associated with mass slaughter"[2] (p. 289). Semelin refers back to what he said at the beginning, that the encounter with such cruelty can produce a

> kind of mental paralysis. However, the attempt to comprehend the process of crossing the threshold into violence would be incomplete if one balked at 'grasping' these phenomena of cruelty [...] It is neither masochism nor voyeurism on the part of the researcher, but just the intuition that, in this terrible act lies one of the keys, if not *the* key to the explosive power of massacre. It is the horror of an act of cruelty which will probably forever remain in the memory of the surviving victim.
>
> (p. 289; author's emphasis)[3]

Semelin goes on to describe the ecstasy of cruelty, what Weisband called the "macabresque." According to him:

> Perpetrators of atrocities can be said to enter [...] delirious episodes, and this metamorphosis can occur all the more easily when it is authorized by society (p. 298). [...] Omnipotence, being able to kill without restraint, can be intoxicating (p. 299). [...] Violent practices seem to be inherent in the human condition [...] partly because they give some pleasure. Humiliating others and worse still, making them suffer, can provide a form of enjoyment: either by sexually possessing their bodies, or by torturing

> their bodies [...] before annihilating them [...] the situation of impunity creates the conditions for becoming drunk on violence. This is the way the perpetrator can feel genuine pleasure, not only at making the victim suffer but by enjoying the all-powerful state over the victim who is completely at his mercy.
>
> (p. 302)

Not only are paranoid-schizoid dynamics built into sovereignty, so is the pleasure of cruelty.

Here Semelin refers to La Fontaine's *The Wolf and the Lamb*, with its famous statement that might makes right. "Might makes right" is the canonical translation, but is not accurate. In the original it is: *La raison du plus fort est toujours la meilleure*. More accurately: the reasoning, the logic, of the strongest is always best. This is necessary to understand the dialogue between the wolf and the lamb. In brief: a wolf finds a lamb drinking from a stream and accuses it of muddying the water. The lamb offers every possible reason why it has not interfered with the wolf's drinking, but the *cruel* wolf rejects every logical argument on the lamb's part, responding with his own twisted logic. When the wolf accuses the lamb of having slandered it a year before, the lamb says it was not even born then. When the wolf says that it must have been his brother, the lamb says that it has no brother. The wolf responds that it must have been someone from the lamb's family. He then carries off the lamb to devour it. In our terms here, the wolf "knows," i.e., believes unshakably, that like the men and dogs that persecute it, so too the lamb. The cruelty of his *persecutory* illogic prevails.

Semelin claims that Sade cites the fable. It seems that there is no direct citation of it in Sade, but rather a kind of symbolic link to the cruel libertine who takes pleasure in his power to make the innocent victim suffer. Does Sade's libertine justify his cruelty by his own persecution, as does the wolf? Even if not, by referring to Sade, Semelin is asking us to peer into the "black hole," and to see the "intense pleasure of delighting in the suffering and humiliating of others" (p. 303), the "ecstasy of total power" (p. 304). Here, we find an aspect of the paranoid-schizoid position that Klein did not elaborate: its potentially intense erotization. (Charny spoke of the pleasure in destructive power.) Returning to the leader's idealized paranoid-schizoid position, and to Freud's idea that the group is held together by shared love for the leader, in promising omnipotence the leader implicitly promises this ecstasy of total power. "Implicitly" because the "promise" is the leader's intuitive understanding of unconscious dynamics. If one imagines La Fontaine's wolf as a genocidal leader, who "explains" why the lamb cannot be innocent, has to be blamed for "contamination" of the water, his logic, in Semelin's words, is "'*grafted*' on to and feeds on" the universal "elemental psychological core, rooted in the *imaginaire* of early childhood ... [that] is at the basis of a process of violence" (p. 50).

Like the wolf's logic, then, Semelin says, "...there is rationality behind the practices of extreme violence, even if this rationality seems delusional to us" (p. 326). In political terms, it "is as if the modern state, viewing itself as a homogenous self, an 'us' imagined on a political ethnic and/or religious basis, necessarily had to build itself against an other to be expelled, if not destroyed" (p. 336). This is the logic of exclusion of the difference which makes identity possible; the logic of the inevitable inclusion of the allegedly excluded. The logic of the delusional rationality that creates the "vampiric" state, which "sucks the lifeblood" out of its own citizens by inciting them to massacre. The vampirism of self-destructive self-preservation. What is a vampire? The living dead.

All these expressions—delusional rationality, self-destructive self-preservation, inclusion of the excluded, living dead, and stabilizing instability—are self-contradictory. There is another self-contradictory state Semelin describes that affects the researcher into genocide. There is always "moral indignation" about the failure of the international community to act to prevent genocide, but simultaneously an understanding of why this is so—the problem of sovereignty. One is torn between universal morality and the realities of international relations (p. 362). "To accept living with this contradiction, we have to develop a kind of paradoxical thinking: one that reasons from the vantage point of antagonistic propositions" (p. 363). To "accept living with this contradiction" is to *think paradoxically*, to be able to reason on the basis of the apparently unreasonable: antagonistic, self-contradictory propositions. The largest implication of all this is that the researcher, motivated to use understanding in order to prevent, comes to the conclusion that prevention is impossible. Semelin puts it this way: "While the researcher cannot exercise any protective responsibility he can at least take on the *responsibility to know and to make known*" (p. 372; author's emphasis).

Perhaps we have gained another piece of knowledge based on self-contradictory propositions. The leader of the genocidal state promises the omnipotence and ecstasy of the paranoid-schizoid position. But the same leader is also a vampire, the living dead. There was a phenomenon described by survivors of the concentration camps of what was called "*musselmänner*," those who had given up all desire to survive, and were a kind of living dead, although without any vampiric ability to sustain themselves on blood. Are these living dead of the camps the inverse of the vampiric leader? The logical endpoint of the genocidal project as a kind of cancer, an autoimmune disorder of the mind and the state?

Notes

1 Moses, p. 15, gave important early examples of proposals to limit state sovereignty.
2 Nonetheless, in Weisband (Chapter 4), we cited Arendt on Eichmann's simultaneous normality and sadism.
3 Moses spoke of victims' "discernment" of perpetrators' hatred, no matter how matter-of-fact they kill.

9 Sovereignty, Cruelty, and Oneness

At the beginning of *Purify and Destroy*, Semelin said that because mass murder is "absolutely mind-boggling," one might be "paralyzed by his subject matter" (p. 6). This could lead to the "cliche of conventional discourse" that genocide is "unthinkable" (p. 7). To counter the cliche he said that "Of course genocide is thinkable—unfortunately it is too thinkable" (p. 6). Nonetheless, "the closer one draws to the fundamental core of human cruelty, the more he is faced with a sort of 'black hole' that resists any sort of understanding via the intellect" (p. 6). And toward the end of the book he said that to live with all the contradictions implicit to genocide—thinkable, incomprehensible—"we have to develop a kind of paradoxical thinking: one that reasons from the vantage point of antagonistic propositions" (p. 363). In the essay on Dylann Roof, I first began to develop the paradoxical concept of normal psychosis, using the concepts from Freud, Klein, and Bion recapitulated here. And in that essay I began to show why deconstructive thinking, precisely the thinking that "reasons from the vantage point of antagonistic propositions," was necessary in order to think the unthinkable. Indeed, that possibility was brought up in the hearing to assess Roof's mental competence to represent himself at sentencing. The prosecutor said that it seemed that Roof had to be either mentally ill or an irredeemable monster, but because one could not decide between them, there must be a "third option," for which there is "no descriptor" (Bass, 2021, p. 305).

To think from the vantage of antagonistic propositions which require the third option for which there is no conventional descriptor, is, for deconstruction, for Derrida, to think the paradoxically undecidable and impossible. We have seen the necessity of this kind of thinking in relation to genocide throughout: self-destructive self-preservation, murderous suicide, delusional rationality. Bauman said that for the Nazis the Jew was the paradoxical outsider insider, the foreigner within (for which there is no descriptor), and hence the "viscous," "oozing," "conceptual Jew,"—"oozing" precisely because of its blurring of accepted oppositions. There is the paradox of sovereignty: it protects genocide. And if genocide is the "black hole" of "human cruelty," "that *resists* any sort of understanding via the intellect" (my emphasis),

DOI: 10.4324/9781003562870-10

then the encounter with that resistance takes us to the undecidable and the impossible.

In 2000 there was a conference in Paris called *Les Etats généraux de la psychanalyse* ("The Estates General of Psychoanalysis," referencing the meeting of the three estates that preceded the French Revolution). Derrida gave a long address there whose subtitle directly addresses the undecidable impossible of our central topic: "The Impossible Beyond of a Sovereign Cruelty." Sovereignty as cruel; cruelty as sovereign—the fundamental logic of genocide. Derrida contended that cruelty itself is one of the "horizons most proper to psychoanalysis" (p. 239), citing many places where Freud adduces a cruelty, an aggression, that cannot be eliminated. If cruelty is endless, without limit (p. 239), then:

> Let us merely ask ourselves whether, yes or no, what is called 'psychoanalysis' does not open up the only way that could allow us, if not to know, if not to think even, at least to interrogate what might be meant by this strange and familiar word 'cruelty' [...] if this irreducible thing in the life of the animate being is indeed the possibility of cruelty (the drive, if you will, of evil for evil, of a suffering that would play at enjoying the suffering of a making-suffer or a making-oneself-suffer for the pleasure of it), then no other discourse—be it theological, metaphysical, genetic, physicalist, cognitivist, and so forth—could open itself up to this hypothesis. They would all be designed to reduce it, exclude it, deprive it of sense. The only discourse that can today claim the thing of psychical suffering as its own affair would indeed be what has been called, for about a century, psychoanalysis.
>
> (pp. 239–240)

Weisband also contended that only psychoanalysis allows one to understand the surplus cruelty that always attends genocide (the "macabresque"). Cruelty was an essential topic for Semelin.

When Derrida speaks of an "impossible *beyond*" of sovereign cruelty, he is of course referring to the "*beyond* of the pleasure principle." If cruelty is irreducible, one might have to see whether its conjunction with the beyond of the pleasure *principle*, the death drive, is also what one cannot go beyond. Or if—crucially—one might "*think*" (my emphasis) an "*impossible* thing, namely, a beyond of the death drive or the drive for sovereign mastery, the beyond of a cruelty, a beyond that would have nothing to do with either drives or principles" (p. 241; my emphasis). To think this impossible beyond of sovereign cruelty *is* to think the impossible beyond genocide. To think the impossible beyond genocide, then, is to *suffer* what Derrida calls the "ordeal of the undecidable" (p. 241). To think the impossible beyond genocide is to suffer, to make oneself suffer—although not for the pleasure of it—but rather to suffer facing the impossible beyond genocide.[1]

If there is no beyond of sovereignty or cruelty, then, says Derrida, they "resist." (Semelin: the black hole of cruelty resists understanding.) They resist any surpassing of them. Genocide resists, resists every hope of "never again," every effort to see it as exceptional, every effort to understand it in the name of prevention—including this one. Weisband had spoken of another resistance, the general resistance of social or political scientists to psychoanalysis. Analogously, Derrida speaks of the larger resistance to psychoanalysis in the world.[2] The world resists the most basic psychoanalytic thought: the larger part of the mind is not conscious; the ego is not master in its own house. Derrida integrates this resistance to psychoanalysis with the question of sovereignty. He says that it is a manifestation of the

> metaphysics of sovereignty (autonomy and omnipotence of the subject-individual or state-freedom, egological will, conscious intentionality). The first gesture of psychoanalysis will have been to explain this sovereignty, to give an account of its ineluctability while aiming to deconstruct its genealogy which passes also by way of cruel murder.
>
> (pp. 243–244)

Freud:

> conflicts of interest between men are settled by the use of violence [...] From the moment at which weapons were introduced, intellectual superiority already began to replace brute muscular strength; but the final purpose of the fight remained the same—one side or the other was to be compelled to abandon his claim or his objection by the damage inflicted on him and by the crippling of his strength. That purpose was most completely achieved if the victor's violence eliminated his opponent permanently—that is to say, killed him
>
> (S.E., 22, 204)

The unquestioned belief in the sovereignty of the state *is* the unquestioned belief in the conscious subject, its autonomy, and omnipotence. As soon as sovereignty becomes unsurpassable, all the dynamics of the murderousness at its origin are at work. According to Freud:

> There was a path that led from violence to right or law [...] Violence could be broken by union, and the power of those who were united now represented law in contrast to the violence of the single individual. Thus we see that right [*Recht*] is the might [*Macht*] of a community.
>
> (22, 205)

The sovereign state, as Freud had already said, prohibits violence in order to monopolize it—in the name of *Recht*, law itself. Might makes right, as in the purported lesson of *The Wolf and the Lamb*.

There is another resistance—the resistance of psychoanalysis to itself. By this Derrida means the resistance of psychoanalysis to undertaking the "interrogation" of sovereign cruelty. He says:

> As I see it, psychoanalysis has not yet undertaken and thus still less succeeded in thinking, penetrating, and changing the axioms of the ethical, the juridical, and the political, notably in those seismic places where the theological phantasm of sovereignty quakes and where the most traumatic, let us say in a still confused manner the most cruel events of our day are being produced.
>
> (p. 244)

To call sovereignty a "theological phantasm" is to understand it as the fantasy of god-like omnipotence, the fantasy of the narcissistic subject, the subject who reacts to difference with primal violence. To say that this fantasy "quakes" where the most cruel events are produced is to say that this is where the paradox of sovereignty, that it protects the most cruel events, is felt. Derrida mentions genocide and crimes against humanity here (p. 244). In Freud's writings there is no mention at all of what we now call the German genocide of the Herero of Southwest Africa or the Turkish genocide of the Armenians, both of which were widely reported in the international press at the time.

The necessary "quaking" of unquestioned sovereignty has a history. Above, Moses (p. 153) referenced Pella in 1925 ("crimes so grave as to justify violating the principle of state sovereignty in the interests of 'restoring the moral order which must reign in the whole of humanity' ") and Mandelstam (p. 155) in 1917 and later (rights do not inhere in states, instead there is "sovereignty of law above the state"; and there are "crimes so grave as to justify violating the principle of state sovereignty in the interests of 'restoring the moral order which must reign in the whole of humanity' "). The 1948 UN Convention Against Genocide in the wake of the Holocaust attempted to establish a worldwide proscription of genocide. But it was also adopted at a time of decolonization, when respect for new nations' sovereignty was a crucial issue. Moreover, there was resistance on the part of some major powers to sign the Convention, because they feared it would leave them open to the charge of genocide. To take only one example, the United States did not sign until 1988. And we have seen that in 1999, Kofi Annan, then Secretary-General of the UN, proposed changing the definition of sovereignty so that it could do justice to individual aspirations to freedom. As above: Two years later the International Commission on Intervention and State Sovereignty went further, stating that "defense of state sovereignty ... does not include any claim of the unlimited power of a state to do what it wants to its own people" (p. 8). Sovereignty implies dual responsibility: to respect the sovereignty of other states and to respect the basic rights of all people in the state (p. 8). This redefinition of state sovereignty changes sovereignty from control to sovereignty as responsibility. In 2005 the doctrine of sovereignty as responsibility was adopted by the General Assembly. A 2019 UN report on what came to be called "Responsibility to Protect" bleakly stated that everything was "moving in the wrong direction." Sovereignty as responsibility is still sovereignty.

Here one might possibly get beyond psychoanalysis' resistance to itself. To change sovereignty as control to sovereignty as responsibility is to move from the paranoid-schizoid to the depressive position. Psychoanalysis (Klein) tells us that there is no depressive position without a paranoid-schizoid position. The depressive position produces extreme anxiety when the good, *idealized* object is integrated with the bad persecutory object, leading to fear of its loss, and consequent regression to the paranoid-schizoid position. To which it is essential to add the possible reintegration of violently excluded *difference*, leading to fear of chaotic loss of control. These are the main reasons why changing sovereignty as control to sovereignty as responsibility can exacerbate cruelty, aggression, and the tendency to genocide. This is not to say that the idea is unjustified, but rather that it needs to be accompanied by an understanding of the resistance it inevitably engenders. This is why Derrida can say that psychoanalysis:

> should have something indispensable and essential not just to say but also to do on this subject [...] The decisive thing that there would be to say and to do on this subject should register the shock wave of one or more psychoanalytic revolutions. Notably on the subject of what is called, therefore, sovereignty and cruelty.
>
> (p. 245)

In *States...*, looking at *Why War?*, the exchange between Einstein and Freud, Derrida says that Einstein's basic points are as true today as they were in 1932. Einstein advocates the establishment of a "legislative and judicial body to settle every conflict arising between nationals" (S.E.22, pp. 199–200). This leads to what Einstein calls his "first axiom: the quest of international security involves the unconditional surrender by every nation, in a certain measure, of its liberty of action, its sovereignty" (22, p. 200). The problem is that an international tribunal does not have at its command the necessary means to enforce its decisions. Derrida:

> force and right (*Macht und Recht*) go hand in hand. Juridical decisions approach the ideal of justice demanded by the human community only to the extent that this community has at its disposal a force of constraint able to command respect for its ideal.
>
> (*States*, p. 252)

Einstein advocates that every nation abandon unconditionally at least a part of its sovereignty and also recognizes that strong psychological factors paralyze efforts toward international justice (p. 252). He speaks of the "*craving for power* which characterizes the governing class in every nation," making it "hostile to any limitation of the national sovereignty" (22, p. 200; my emphasis). Derrida here sees Einstein agreeing with Freud on the irreducibility of aggression. No doubt. But this is where we add that the hostility to any limitation of sovereignty is motivated by the anxieties of the depressive position and by fear of chaotic loss of control. Derrida comments that

> Einstein advances at this point a hypothesis that anticipates the direction of what will be Freud's reply, namely, that of a cruelty drive (that is, basically a death drive), which, without being reduced to it, is coupled with the drive for power (*Bemächtigungstrieb*) that has such an original place in *Beyond the Pleasure Principle*. What could one do with an irreducible death drive and an invincible drive for power in a politics and a law that would be progressive, that is to say, confident, as during the Enlightenment, in some perfectibility?
>
> (*States,* p. 252)

In other words, what if a death drive and a drive for power are the limits of progress? The irreducible obstacles to prevention of genocide?

Einstein goes further on this point. He says that "man has within him a lust for hatred and destruction" (22, p. 201); "it is a comparatively easy task to call it into play and raise it to the power of a collective psychosis" (p. 201). When Einstein speaks of a "collective psychosis" I think he means what Freud, following Le Bon, meant in *Group Psychology.* The "lust for hatred and destruction" in every individual can become the regressed identity of the collectivity itself. Adding to Freud on group identification with the leader, we have contended that such a collective psychosis is the result of identification with the leader's idealized paranoid-schizoid position.

All of this leads Einstein to ask the *impossible*, but necessary, question we have encountered all along (Waller, Charny): "Is it possible to control man's mental evolution so as to make him proof against the psychoses of hate and destructiveness?" (p. 201) Einstein is careful to note that his question about evolution does not simply concern what might be considered the least evolved portion of humanity: "Here I am thinking by no means only of the so-called uncultured masses. Experience proves that it is rather the so-called 'Intelligentzia' that is most apt to yield to these disastrous collective suggestions" (p. 201).[3]

Turning to Freud in *Why War?*, Derrida makes a summary statement:

> If the drive for power or the cruelty drive is irreducible, older, more ancient than the principles (the pleasure principle or the reality principle [...]), then no politics will be able to eradicate it. Politics can only domesticate it, differ and defer it, learn to negotiate, compromise indirectly but without illusion with it, and it is this indirection, this differing/deferring detour, this

> system of differantial relays and delays that will dictate Freud's at once optimistic and pessimistic politics.
>
> (*States*, p. 252)

Anyone familiar with Derrida's work will recognize his essential "concept" of *différance*: simultaneous differing in space and deferring in time. Freud will indeed speak of indirect ways of dealing with irreducible sovereign cruelty. Derrida links this to another concept of Freud's that he thinks is inadequately appreciated: the *Bemächtigungstrieb*, the drive for power.[4] We have just seen Derrida allude to it in his discussion of Einstein in *Why War?*, especially because of its relation to the death drive in *Beyond the Pleasure Principle*. In his reading of *Beyond*... in *The Post Card*, Derrida had already called the *Bemächtigungstrieb* the "driven of the drive," the force that makes the drive a drive—a kind of "meta-drive." He now expands his sense of the *Bemächtigungstrieb:*

> Indissociable from that of *Bewaltigung* (exercise of power, ascendancy, or possession, movement of appropriation, etc.), there would thus be the concept of a drive for power—that is to say, of the capacitation, of the "I can" or "I may." This drive for power no doubt indicates, before and beyond any principle, before and beyond any power even (the principle being the power, the sovereignty of the power), one of the places where the Freudian psychoanalytic discourse is articulated with juridical and political questions in general, with all that concerns the new givens, today, of this double problematic of sovereignty and cruelty.
>
> (p. 258)[5]

When Derrida speaks of the "capacitation" of the "I can" or "I may" one might wonder whether he is contradicting himself on the "first gesture of psychoanalysis": the deconstruction of the autonomous, conscious ego. But I think he is making a basic psychoanalytic point. The belief in the autonomous, conscious ego that says I can or I may is the manifestation of the drive for power. It is the blind force, the drivenness of drives, that allows the sovereign state to say it can, it may, it has the autonomous right, to kill its own citizens in any form (death penalty, war, genocide). This is why Derrida says that:

> so long as a coherent psychoanalytic discourse will not have treated (and to my knowledge it has not yet done so) the problem of the death penalty and of sovereignty in general, of the sovereign power of the state over the life and death of citizens, this will make manifest a double resistance, both that of the world to psychoanalysis and that of psychoanalysis to itself as to the world, of psychoanalysis to psychoanalysis as being-in-the-world.
>
> (p. 262)

Derrida then reemphasizes the relation between "might and right" (*Macht und Recht*) he found in Einstein's point about the force necessary to curtail sovereignty. For Freud, as we know, "right [*Recht*] is the might [*Macht*] of a community" as the result of primal murder. Without referring directly to Freud, Derrida echoes him when he says: "Right becomes the power or the violence of the community that, by *monopolizing* force, protects itself against individual violence. Force against force, deferred economy of force: this is what makes right" (p. 270). In other words, force is irreducible. It can be redirected into another form of force, the force of law itself. But this means that the power, the sovereignty of the law contains within it cruelty and aggression, such that law itself can command murder. (This is why Derrida puts so much emphasis on the death penalty.) "Making very frequent use of the words 'cruelty,' 'aggression drive,' 'hatred drive,' and 'death drive,' [Freud] denounces an illusion: that of an eradication of the cruelty drives and the drives for power and sovereignty" (p. 270).

This where I wish Freud had said something about Einstein on collective psychosis. If it is an illusion to eradicate the drives for power and sovereignty, would it not also be an illusion to eradicate the possibility of the collective, normalized psychosis of genocide? There is a hint in this direction, when Derrida writes:

> Freudian philosophy of culture, of civilization, or history [...] always comes back to this motif: teleology of a progress by indirect displacement and restriction of the forces of the drives, thus of a cruelty that, indestructible in any event, produces war or murder and may lead, the word is Freud's, to the 'extermination' of the enemy.
>
> (p. 272)[6]

What does "may lead" mean here? That Freud *was* aware of the exterminations of the Herero and the Armenians in his time, to say nothing of all the previous exterminations of history? Or that he sees this as a possibility, but has not registered its actuality?

Responding to Einstein on what psychoanalysis might offer to affect cruelty and aggression indirectly, Freud adduces the life drive, Eros:

> Our mythological theory of instincts makes it easy for us to find a formula for *indirect* methods of combating war. If willingness to engage in war is an effect of the destructive instinct, the most obvious plan will be to bring Eros, its antagonist, into play against it.
>
> (22, p. 212; Freud's emphasis)

Derrida comments:

> Indirection, the ruse of the detour (*Umweg*), consists [...] in bringing into play the antagonistic force of Eros, love and the love of life, against the

> death drive. There is thus a contrary to the cruelty drive, even if the latter knows no end. There is an opposable term, even if there is not a term that puts an end to the opposition.
>
> (p. 272)

In speaking of bringing Eros into play against the destructive instinct, Freud forgets himself in two ways which compromise Derrida's comment about a contrary to the cruelty drive.

First, in *Civilization and Its Discontents*, Freud had written:

> Not merely is [the] stranger in general unworthy of my love; I must honestly confess that he has more claim to my hostility and even my hatred. He seems not to have the least trace of love for me and shows me not the slightest consideration. If it will do him any good he has no hesitation in injuring me, nor does he ask himself whether the amount of advantage he gains bears any proportion to the extent of the harm he does to me. Indeed, he need not even obtain an advantage; if he can satisfy any sort of desire by it, he thinks nothing of jeering at me, insulting me, slandering me and showing his superior power; and the more secure he feels and the more helpless I am, the more certainly I can expect him to behave like this to me.
>
> (21, p. 110)[7]

Consistent with his earlier remarks about hate older than love (in "Instincts and Their Vicissitudes") and about primal violence against racial difference (in *Group Psychology),* Freud thinks there is primal violence and even gratuitous cruelty between "strangers"—those different from each other. Continuing in the same passage, which is a commentary on "love thy neighbor as thyself," Freud says:

> If [the stranger] behaves differently, if he shows me consideration and forbearance as a stranger, I am ready to treat him in the same way, in any case and quite apart from any precept. Indeed, *if* this grandiose commandment had run 'Love thy neighbour as thy neighbour loves thee', I should not take exception to it.
>
> (p. 110 [my emphasis])

In other words, the best one might hope for is a *quid pro quo* which depends upon an unlikely "if." Perhaps Freud does not want to say to Einstein that to "bring Eros," the "antagonist" of the death drive, "into play against it" requires bargaining.

Second, Freud does not mention his own conception of Eros as a "mischief maker" that raises tension levels by introducing "fresh vital differences." This is why he also speaks of a "struggle against Eros." Paradoxically, there is a necessary cruelty to Eros. To "love thy neighbor [the stranger] as thyself," can both be vitally necessary and inflict increased tension on oneself. To love the stranger/neighbor who could be the victim of genocide is to withstand the tension that the psyche primally tends to discharge. Responsibility to protect is cruel, the ethical cruelty of enduring the anxieties of the depressive position and fear of chaotic loss of control. This is why we have said that to think the impossible beyond is to "suffer the *ordeal* of the undecidable." It is undecidable that Eros is the contrary of cruelty. It is; but it comports its own cruelty. Derrida:

> It is in this place that is difficult to delimit, the space of undecidability and thus of decision opened up by the discontinuity of the indirect, that the transformation to come of ethics, law, and politics should take into account psychoanalytic knowledge.
>
> (p. 273)

While Freud does not refer to his own more paradoxical remarks about Eros, he does refer to another "undecidable," the inevitable mixture of Eros and the death drive: "Neither of these instincts is any less essential than the other; the phenomena of life arise from the concurrent *or* mutually opposing action of both" (22, 209, [my emphasis]). I emphasize "or" here to make the point that if Eros and the death drive can act concurrently *or* in opposition, the opposition between them is not absolute. (This is why in his reading of *Beyond the Pleasure Principle* in *The Post Card* Derrida speaks of life-death.) How might this affect the interrogation of sovereignty and cruelty? In Freud's own terms, there could be no absolute bringing "into play" of Eros against the death drive, because they do act concurrently or in opposition. (In *Beyond the Pleasure Principle,* Freud had spoken of the "vacillating rhythm" of the life and death drives and of the anabolistic *and* catabolistic aspect of each [18, 41].) As Derrida has emphasized, Freud speaks of indirection here. This would have to be even more the case if there is a cruelty to Eros, so that the cruel death drive can appear to operate *against* cruelty by relieving the tension of Eros. Perpetrators of genocide often see themselves as ethical heroes. Unconsciously they are protecting their group against the quasi-traumatic experience of the tension of Eros.

Freud then returns to his basic idea from *Totem and Taboo* and *Group Psychology* that "violence [is] overcome by the transference of power to a larger unity, which is held together by emotional ties between its members" (22, 205). But "attempts are made by certain of the rulers to set themselves above the prohibitions which apply to everyone—they seek, that is, to go back from a dominion of law to a dominion of violence" (22, 206). Moreover, as we have already seen, "law was originally brute violence and ... even to-day it cannot do without the support of violence" (22, 209). In *Group Psychology*, Freud said that the emotional ties between members of the group are their identifications with the idealized leader. Hence, there can there can be identification with the leader's "dominion of violence," his paranoid-schizoid dynamics. And if law itself contains violence, then this identification can lead to—referring back to Einstein—the "collective psychosis" of paradoxical lawful violence (e.g., the Nuremberg laws, Jim Crow laws).

Freud suggests that to counter the violence of rulers

> more care should be taken than hitherto to educate an upper stratum of men with independent minds, not open to intimidation and eager in the pursuit of truth, whose business it would be to give direction to the dependent masses.
>
> (22, 212)

Is this a question of education? When Einstein asked if it was possible to control man's mental evolution to make him "proof against the psychoses of hate and destructiveness," he was careful to note that it is the "so-called 'Intelligentzia' that is most apt to yield to these disastrous collective suggestions." Einstein here adds something to Freud on groups and leaders. His member of the "intelligentsia" yields to disastrous *collective* suggestion. Education is not proof against the psychoses of hate and destructiveness, because paranoid-schizoid mechanisms are an inherent part of man's "mental evolution." The history of genocide is one of intelligent leaders understanding what Einstein called the collective psychoses of hate and destructiveness,[8] and of making themselves the idealized incarnation of it in the name of ethics and law, thereby intensifying group identification, as Freud might suggest.

Freud does deal with the question of evolution raised by Einstein, although without seeming to answer Einstein's question about the possible control of evolution. As Derrida noted, for Freud progress depends upon the indirect displacement and redirection of the drives. Consistent with his arguments in *Civilization and Its Discontents,* Freud writes:

> For incalculable ages mankind has been passing through a process of evolution of culture. (Some people, I know, prefer to use the term 'civilization'.) We owe to that process the best of what we have become, as well as a good part of what we suffer from. Though its causes and beginnings are obscure and its outcome uncertain, some of its characteristics are easy to perceive. It may perhaps be leading to the extinction of the human race, for in more than one way it impairs the sexual function; uncultivated races and backward strata of the population are already multiplying more rapidly than highly cultivated ones. The process is perhaps comparable to the domestication of certain species of animals and it is undoubtedly accompanied by physical alterations; but we are still unfamiliar with the notion that the evolution of civilization is an organic process of this kind. The psychical modifications that go along with the process of civilization are striking and unambiguous. They consist in a progressive displacement of instinctual aims and a restriction of instinctual impulses.
>
> (22, 214)

I have deliberately quoted this passage in full, so as not to bypass Freud's eugenicist comment about uncultivated races multiplying more rapidly than cultivated ones. The extreme irony here is that, today, the extinction of the human race is indeed possible. It is lodged in the technology of the "highly cultivated." One cannot say "races" because such technological advance (and concomitant environmental destruction) is certainly human but not racial. Freud had already said that "From the moment at which weapons were introduced, intellectual superiority already began to replace brute muscular strength." And he had already seen the possibility of extermination of "enemies" due to the technological advances of warfare. This is why I think that Freud is right to consider that the "evolution of civilization" might be an "organic process." When he compares this to the physical alterations of domesticated animals, it is unclear whether he means that they reproduce less than the undomesticated, as the context suggests, or that as their instincts are curbed they change bodily, or possibly both. His statement about the evolution of culture producing what we "suffer from" is a direct echo of his idea that inhibition or internalization of aggression is responsible for the existence of the super-ego, which can be as *cruel* as the id. And while Freud would probably consider Eros, the life drive, as largely responsible for "the best of what we have become," he did not consider his own idea that it differentiates and raises tension levels, and is thus a mischief-maker. We have placed great emphasis on Klein's idea of the depressive position, of *responsibility* for one's aggression. And we know that the depressive position, like Eros, contains its own tensions, its own anxieties. Integrating Freud and Klein, responsibility for aggression is a tension-raising, differentiating process. Responsibility to protect entails suffering. But if man's "mental evolution" (perhaps comparable to a domesticating, organic process) is to counter genocide and ecocide, it cannot evade this suffering. Might internalization of this suffering modify evolution itself?

Freud metaphorically alludes to something like this when he speaks of "we pacifists" who have a "constitutional intolerance of war" (22, 214). The phrase "constitutional intolerance of war" does not sound psychoanalytic. It makes intolerance of war something like an allergy ("lactose intolerance"), a bodily process. But to push the metaphor, for Freud pacifists have an autoimmune condition that the rest of destructive humanity does not. Which again suggests continuity between the body and culture/civilization. Might this allergy to war be the result of suffering the tensions of the depressive position and Eros? Might the impossible beyond of sovereignty, cruelty, and genocide, be a pandemic of this allergy, the suffering, the ordeal of these tensions? Might this be a crucial adaptation for man's evolution? At the very least we know that without something like this Responsibility to Protect is an inevitable failure.

Along these lines, Derrida makes an important distinction between sovereignty and unconditionality. On one hand, he says, "Both of these escape absolutely, like the absolute itself, all relativism" (*Rogues*, p. xiv). On the other, "... through the experience that lets itself be affected by what or who comes [*(ce) qui vient*], by what happens or by who happens by, by *the other to come,* a certain unconditional renunciation of sovereignty is required a priori" (p. xiv). I think that what Derrida means here is that if one is open to what is entirely other than what one expects, because expectation conforms to one's presuppositions, then one has to have foregone sovereignty. He continues: "... [this] presupposes that we think at once the unforeseeability of an event that is necessarily without horizon, the singular coming of the other, and as a result a *weak* force" (p. xiv). If sadism and cruelty are the *Bemächtigungstrieb,* the drive to power that controls difference and otherness, then, Derrida is telling us, difference and otherness themselves cannot have the force of the *Bemächtigungstrieb.* Hence, their force is weak. Too weak? Is the paranoid-schizoid position stronger than the depressive position? The death drive stronger than Eros? Freud's thought about primal narcissistic violence against racial difference suggests it, as does the perennial nature of genocide. Could a "pandemic" of the "constitutional intolerance" of "war," of suffering the anxieties of the depressive position and the tension of Eros, be such a weak force?

This would affect, or "infect," the power of the autonomous self, or the sovereign state. Derrida says more about autonomy and sovereignty, calling it *ipse:*

> By *'ipséité'* I thus wish to suggest some "I can," or at least the power that gives itself its own law, its force of law, its self representation, the sovereign and reappropriating gathering of self [...] Before any sovereignty of the State, of the Nation-State, of the monarch, or in democracy, of the people, *ipseity* names a principle of legitimate sovereignty, the accredited or recognized supremacy of a power or a force
>
> (*R*, pp. 11–12)

"Ipseity" is then an expansion of the idea of the force implicit to any "I can, I have the right to." There are two very difficult consequences of this idea. First: There is "The law of a terrifying and suicidal autoimmunity [...] a gyrating coincidence between force and right, force and justice, force and the the reason of the strongest" (*R*, p. 18). Second: If "I have the right to" means "I have the force to," it also means "I am free to" (*R*, p.23). The state has the right to, has the force to, is free to commit genocide. Dylann Roof did not doubt that he had the right, the force, the freedom to initiate a race war. In other words, not only does sovereignty protect genocide, so does the freedom of democracy. This is why Derrida says:

> There is something paradigmatic in this autoimmune suicide: fascist and Nazi totalitarianisms came into power [...] through formally normal and formally democratic electoral processes [...] When they are assured of an arithmetic majority, the worst enemies of democratic freedom can present themselves as the most democratic of all.
>
> (*R*, p. 33)

If all of this is related to what Derrida has called the "first gesture of psychoanalysis," i.e., the delimitation of the supposedly free conscious subject, the ego, *ipse*, then he can also ask: "What can a bygone psychoanalysis or one that is still to come tell us about democracy?" (*R*, p. 54).

Pursuing the question, he intensifies its relation to psychoanalysis:

> What psychoanalysts call more or less complacently the unconscious remains, it seems to me, one of the privileged sources, one of the vitally mortal and mortally vital reserves or resources, for this implacable law of the self-destructive conservation of the 'subject' or of egological ipseity [...] without auto-immunity there would be neither psychoanalysis nor what psychoanalysis calls the 'unconscious.' Not to mention, therefore, the 'death drive,' the cruelty of 'primary sadism or masochism'—or even of what we just as complacently call 'consciousness'.
>
> ([*conscience*], *R*, p.55)

Note the paradoxical phrases used to describe autoimmunity: vitally mortal, mortally vital. This is the life and death drives acting in opposition *or* in conjunction, vacillating. And note the paradoxical phrase self-destructive conservation of the subject. The sovereign state, modeled on the autonomous subject, *can* engage in the self-destructive self-preservation of genocide. Derrida is making clear that autoimmunity is intrinsic to the power of the supposedly free, autonomous ego or the state. He lists the structurally autoimmune concepts of death drive and primary sado-masochism. The entire question of conscience itself, once understood in Freudian terms as an id-driven, *cruel* super-ego, can make the self-destructive self-preservation of genocide an ethical obligation. If all of these are essential psychoanalytic concepts, then, yes, "without auto-immunity there would be no psychoanalysis" or "the unconscious." In a strong concluding statement, Derrida writes:

> by speaking in just this way of autoimmunity, I specifically wanted to consider all these processes of, so to speak, normal and normative perversion quite apart from the authority of representative consciousness, of the I, the self, and ipseity. This was also the only way, it seemed to me, of taking into account within politics what psychoanalysis once called the unconscious.
>
> (*R*, pp. 109–110)

Normative perversion—normal psychosis—the processes embedded *in* ipseity, in consciousness, but not *of* consciousness.

Ipse as the self implies oneness: one is oneself. Semelin spoke about genocide in relation to the search for "an essentialized self," an identity purified of the difference that constitutes it (p. 27). He called this "the rage of Oneness" (p. 33), and likened it to paranoia. (Freud: the purified pleasure ego hates and seeks to destroy what it has projected.) In *Archive Fever* Derrida addressed this issue in the following sentence:

> *L'un se garde de l'autre*. The one guards against/keeps some of the other. It protects *itself* from the other, but, in the movement of this jealous violence, it comprises in itself, thus guarding it, the self-otherness or self-difference [...] which makes it One. The 'One differing, deferring from itself' [...] It violates and does violence to itself, but it also institutes itself as violence [...] Self determination as violence. *L'un se garde de l'autre pour se faire violence (because* it makes itself violence and *so as* to make itself violence).
>
> (*AF*, p.78)

If there is no oneness without the other, if oneness depends upon the other, depends upon having the other as part of oneself, then oneness is necessarily violence to itself. Autoimmunity is the ability to protect itself against this violence, oneness has to become violent. The autoimmunity of violence against the other is inextricably linked to violence against oneself. The self-destructive conservation of egological ipseity. In *The Politics of Friendship, a propos* of Schmitt on the essential role of the enemy, Derrida extends these ideas. Describing what he calls one of the subterranean themes of this essay: how the One divides and opposes itself, opposes itself by posing itself, represses and violates the difference it carries within itself, wages war, *wages war on itself,* itself becoming war *[se fait la guerre] frightens itself, itself becoming fear [se fait peur],* and *does violence to itself, itself becoming violence [se fait violence],* transforms itself into frightened violence in guarding itself from the other, for it *guards itself from, and in, the other [il se garde de l'autre],* always, Him, the One, the One different from itself[9] (p. 109; translator's interpolations).

Derrida has added war and fear to his original formulation from *Archive Fever.* This "rage of Oneness" is both the logic and the emotion of genocide. The fear Derrida speaks of is the anxiety about the persecutory object that is oneself, paranoid-schizoid anxiety. Genocide is war motivated by this anxiety.

Sovereignty as *ipse* is always potentially frightened, enraged, cruel, violent. It is the embodiment of might makes right. In *The Beast and the Sovereign* Derrida further explicates the essential lawlessness of sovereignty. Referring to Schmitt's definition of the sovereign as "the exception," Derrida writes that:

> sovereignty is a certain power to *give,* to *make,* but also to *suspend* the law; it is the exceptional right to place oneself above right, the right to non-right ... which runs the risk of carrying the human sovereign above the human, toward divine omnipotence (which will moreover most often have grounded the principle of sovereignty in its sacred and theological origin) and, because of this arbitrary suspension or rupture of right, runs the risk of making the sovereign look like the most brutal beast who respects nothing, scorns the law, immediately situates himself above the law, at a distance from the law ... Being-outside-the-law can, no doubt (and this is the figure

> of sovereignty), take the form of the Law itself, of the origin of laws, the guarantor of laws, as though the Law, with a capital L, the condition of the law, were before, above, and therefore outside the law … but being-outside-the-law can also, on the other hand (and this is the figure of what is most often understood by animality or bestiality) … situate the place where the law does not appear, or is not respected, or gets violated. These modes of being-outside-the-law (be it the mode of what is called the beast, be it that of the criminal …) be it [that] of the sovereign himself—these different modes of being-outside-the-law can seem to be heterogeneous among themselves, or even apparently heterogeneous to the law, but the fact remains, sharing this common being-outside-the-law, beast, criminal, and sovereign have a troubling resemblance: they call on each other and recall each other … there is between sovereign, criminal and beast a sort of obscure and fascinating complicity, or even a worrying mutual attraction … all three of them, the animal, the criminal, and the sovereign, are outside the law …
>
> (pp. 16–17)[10]

This passage recapitulates the dynamics of genocide. Sovereignty as omnipotence is sovereignty as divine. We have seen that the omnipotent one true god who gives the law, also commands genocide as its law. Sovereignty is for Foucault the right to kill, for Freud intrinsically violent, murderous. Thus, the "bestiality" of sovereignty, the bestiality of genocide. The lawfulness of bestiality (instinct and ethics as in Diamond). The paradoxical lawfulness of criminality.

But the sovereign god-criminal-beast also protects.

> The word *protection* bears the whole burden of the political, i.e. the insurance contract between scared or terrorized subjects to delegate to the state or the sovereign the charge of protecting them when they cannot protect themselves […] 'I protect you' means for the state, I oblige you, you are my subject.
>
> (*B&S,* pp. 42–43; author's emphasis)

Himmler's famous words state this clearly: "we had the duty to our people to do it, to destroy this people who wanted to destroy us." Genocide gives an obvious twist to the idea of protection, as is also clear from Himmler's words. The paranoid-schizoid dynamics of the sovereign make it necessary to have its subjects believe that they need protection, even when they don't. The one makes itself fear, as in Derrida's expression. But this is always possible, given the universality of paranoid-schizoid dynamics and the narcissistically violent response to difference. Again, this is why accusation in the mirror works, as is also clear from Himmler's words. And once it works, the sovereign's bestiality and criminality is godlike, idealized. Bauman noted that the more Jews were vilified, the more Hitler was idolized.

> Which is also why any form of sovereignty bears all these risks.
>
> a certain modernity has begun to question, to undermine, to put into crisis nation-state sovereignty. Every time one refers to to the universality of human rights (beyond the rights of man and citizen), every time one invokes the recent concept [...] of crime against humanity or genocide, in order to implement an international right or even an international penal tribunal [...] every time one militates for the *universal* abolition of the death penalty, etc., then one is calling into question the principle and the authority of the sovereignty of the nation-state, and doing so in the name of man, the right of man, the proper of man [...] all these agencies might well be invoking another sovereignty, the sovereignty of man himself.
>
> (*B&S,* pp. 70–71; author's emphasis)

We have already seen that Responsibility to Protect protected state sovereignty; hence its failure. Protection of the sovereignty of man himself, even in the well-intentioned protection of basic human rights, does not take into account the "impossible beyond of sovereign cruelty," which is also the "proper of man." Derrida calls for "...a *slow and differentiated* deconstruction of ... the dominant, classical concept of nation-state sovereignty..." (*B&S,* p. 75; author's emphasis). But without a slow, differentiated (weak) deconstruction of the dominant concept of the subject, *ipse,* Oneness, that is, without taking into account the psychoanalytic understanding of man, sovereignty will remain untouched. As Derrida says: "**...**we really do have to take into account a logic of the unconscious that ought to forbid any immediate certainty as to the consciousness of freedom that all responsibility presupposes..." (p. 119).

Concluding Remarks

In my introduction, I alluded to the book *Annihilating Difference: The Anthropology of Genocide,* edited by Alexander Hinton. As I briefly said there, Hinton's title alone can summarize much of what we have tried to develop here. His introductory essay also captures many of our points: "... uncertainty about identity often leads perpetrators to inscribe difference upon the bodies of their victims" (p. 5).[11] Uncertainty about identity is the auto-immunity of Oneness. The word "inscribe" implies something like a tattoo, an incision on the body that marks it. Capturing the group process of creating the "foreigner within" upon whose body difference is inscribed, Hinton writes:

> Genocides are distinguished by a process of 'othering' in which the boundaries of an imagined community are reshaped in such a manner that a previously 'included' group (albeit included only tangentially) is ideologically recast (almost always in dehumanizing rhetoric) as being outside the community, as a threatening and dangerous 'other'—whether racial, political, ethnic, religious, economic, and so on—that must be annihilated.
>
> (p. 6)

The dehumanization of a previously included group is the problem of "the foreigner within." "Boundaries of an imagined community" suggests the problem of the fantasy of an impermeable border whose very existence is due to its (intolerable) porousness. Hinton analyzes "dehumanizing rhetoric" in terms of "value laden binary oppositions" such as us/them, normal/abnormal, human/subhuman, pure/ impure, and law/uncontrolled (pp. 8–9). "If all human beings are born with a propensity to distinguish difference, modern societies are distinguished by the degree to which such differences are reified. In other words, modernity thrives on the essentialization of difference" (p. 12). Essentialization of difference depends upon its reconfiguration as value laden binary oppositions taken as concretely real, the imposition of fantasy upon reality.

And not only modernity. In Hinton's words, the *human* propensity to distinguish difference, to register it, is itself an "inscription" that is both vital and tension-raising (Freud's Eros). A death drive will always "struggle" (Freud's word) against it, projecting it onto (Freud) or into (Klein) the other, violently creating an essential opposition demanding autoimmune purification and destruction. The universality of genocide speaks to this process as basic to "the unconscious."

All my previous work on the disavowal, the registration and repudiation, of difference was derived from Freud on fetishism, and from Freud's final thoughts about fetishism and disavowal as models for basic unconscious processes. Genocide as the *annihilation* of difference is the most violent expression of these dynamics: the registration (Eros) and repudiation (death drive) of difference replaced by the oppositions of the paranoid-schizoid position (idealized/persecutory), with all the self-preservative self-destruction that implies. This is why there is a necessary integration of psychoanalytic and deconstructive thought to understand genocide. Both contain key ways of thinking difference and violence.

Notes

1 Keval had already made an analogous point:

> The challenge of psychoanalysis is to square up to the many faces of racism, and to do so not with the aim of eliminating this type of *cruelty* but to interrogate the psychic investments and the complex alliances that exist between the forces of reason and racism.
>
> (p. 120; my emphasis)

2 Freud, of course, spent a lifetime dealing with this resistance. More technically, in a paper called "The Resistances to Psychoanalysis," he spoke about its derivation from medicine and philosophy, and about the way it is foreign to both, occupying a third position between them. Using Bauman's image, one might say that psychoanalysis oozes between medicine and philosophy.

3 In Kiernan (Chapter 1), we discussed Marcus on why leaders' use of "Accusation in the Mirror," the attribution of one's own genocidal intent to its victim works, due to the "meeting of the minds" between leaders and followers, what Marcus called the "inconvenient insight" of an unconscious process.

4 In Weisband (Chapter 4), we cited two places where Freud speaks of a *Bemächtigungstrieb*, a drive for power, translated as "instinct for mastery" in the *Standard Edition*. In *Three Essays on the Theory of Sexuality* Freud writes:

> the impulse of cruelty arises from the instinct for mastery and appears at a period of sexual life at which the genitals have not yet taken over their later role. It then dominates a phase of sexual life which we shall later describe as a pregenital organization.
>
> (7, 193)

Again, in "Instincts and Their Vicissitudes," Freud says that at the

> stage of the pregenital sadistic-anal organization, the striving for the object appears in the form of an urge for mastery (*Bemächtigungstrieb*), to which injury or annihilation of the object is a matter of indifference. Love in this form and at this preliminary stage is hardly to be distinguished from hate in its attitude towards the object.
>
> (14, pp. 138–139)

Clearly, as Derrida says, the *Bemächtigungstrieb* is linked to cruelty. Then, in *Beyond the Pleasure Principle, a propos* of the fort/da game, and his interpretation that the child is playing at his mother's departure and return, Freud writes:

> On an unprejudiced view one gets an impression that the child turned his experience into a game from another motive. At the outset, he was in a passive situation—he was overpowered by the experience; but, by repeating it, unpleasurable though it was, as a game, he took on an active part. These efforts might be put down to an instinct for mastery that was acting independently of whether the memory was in itself pleasurable or not.
>
> (18, 16)

Here Freud envisages a repetition of the unpleasurable (the mother's departure) independent of the pleasure principle. The link between these passages is in Freud's discussion of sadism and the death drive toward the end of *Beyond*...:

> Is it not plausible to suppose that this sadism is in fact a death instinct which, under the influence of the narcissistic libido, has been forced away from the ego and has consequently only emerged in relation to the object?
>
> (18, 54)

This point depends upon Freud's idea that aggression is the result of directing the self-destructive death drive outward. The forerunner of this point is the purified pleasure ego, which projects unpleasure outward onto the object which it then hates and seeks to destroy: purify and destroy...

5 This is also one of the places where Derrida on Freud on power and sovereignty is to be articulated with Foucault on power and sovereignty.

6 We cited Freud on extermination of the enemy in Bauman, above.

7 Freud rather dismissively refers to his previous discussions of the "narcissism of minor differences" (cited above in Bauman) and of racial difference in relation to this passage:

> I once discussed the phenomenon that it is precisely communities with adjoining territories, and related to each other in other ways as well, who are engaged in

> constant feuds and in ridiculing each other—like the Spaniards and Portuguese, for instance, the North Germans and South Germans, the English and Scotch, and so on.1 I gave this phenomenon the name of 'the narcissism of minor differences', a name which does not do much to explain it. We can now see that it is a convenient and relatively harmless satisfaction of the inclination to aggression, by means of which cohesion between the members of the community is made easier.
>
> (21, 114)

He seems to have forgotten that both times he referred to primal hostility and violence. Semelin, above, addressed the psychoanalytic topic of stranger anxiety.

8 This is the logic of "accusation in the mirror."

9 The reader may recognize "the One different from itself" as Heraclitus' *hen heautoi diapherein,* a phrase of evident importance to Derrida in this context, which is also important in his earlier essay *"Différance"* (in *Margins—Of Philosophy*, p. 22). It suggests that this pre-Socratic formulation of Oneness constituted by difference is precisely what I am calling the logic that genocide wages war against. Recall Bauman on adiaphoristic action.

10 Above, in Kiernan, we cited August Bebel who called the German genocide of the Herero "bestial." The question of beast, sovereign, and criminal takes us back to the question of the xenophobic chimps with whom we share most of our DNA.

11 In Bauman and Weisband, above, we cited Holslag, who makes a similar point about power and inscription on the body:

> Power over the body is of special importance here. It is, in the most literal sense, the ultimate power one has over another. This power goes further than bureaucratic and institutional power; it is the power over personhood. In this sense violence is the ultimate method of making baby-grammar physical, tangible, visible. The hegemony of ideas is not just internalized in the minds of perpetrators and even the victimized group, but even more, it becomes (literally) inscribed in the body.
>
> (pp. 103–104)

Bibliography

Arendt, H. (1977). *Eichmann in Jerusalem*. New York: Penguin Books.

Bartov, O. (2018). *Anatomy of a Genocide*. New York: Simon and Schuster.

Bass, A. (2000). *Difference and Disavowal: The Trauma of Eros*. Stanford, CA: Stanford University Press.

Bass, A. (2006). *Interpretation and Difference: The Strangeness of Care*. Stanford, CA: Stanford University Press.

Bass, A. (2018). *Fetiishism, Psychoanalysis, and Philosophy: The Iridescent Thing*. London: Routledge.

Bass, A. (2021). Murderous Racism as Normal Psychosis: The Case of Dylann Roof. *Journal of the American Psychoanalytic Association*. 69: 291–313.

Bauman, Z. (2000). *Modernity and the Holocaust*. Ithaca: Cornell University Press.

Bion, W.R. (1957). Differentiation of the Psychotic from the Non-psychotic Personalities. *International Journal of Psychoanalysis*. 38: 266–275.

Charny, I. (1982). *How Can We Commit the Unthinkable?* Boulder, CO: Westview Press.

Derrida, J. (1982). *Différance*. In *Margins: Of Philosophy*. (A. Bass, trans.) Chicago, IL: University of Chicago Press.

Derrida, J. (1995). *Archive Fever*. (E. Prenowitz, trans.). Chicago, IL: University of Chicago Press.

Derrida, J. (2005a). *The Politics of Friendship*. (G. Collins, trans.). New York: Verso.

Derrida, J. (2005b). *Rogues*. (Brault, P-A. and Naas, M. trans.). Stanford, CA: Stanford University Press.

Derrida, J. (2011). *The Beast and the Sovereign*. (G. Bennington, trans.). Chicago, IL: University of Chicago Press.

Diamond, J. (1993). *The Third Chimpanzee. The Evolution and Future of the Human Animal*. New York: Harper Perennial.

Foucault, M. (2003). *'Society Must Be Defended.' Lectures at the College de France 1975–1976*. (D. Macey, trans.). New York: Picador.

Freud, S. (1905). *Three Essays on the Theory of Sexuality. Standard Edition of the Complete Psychological Works of Sigmund Freud*. (J. Strachey, gen.ed.). London: Hogarth.

Freud, S. (1911). *Formulations of the Two Principles of Mental Functioning*. S.E. 12.

Freud, S. (1913). *Totem and Taboo*. S.E. 13.

Freud, S. (1915a). *Instincts and their Vicissitudes*. S.E. 14

Freud, S. (1915b). *Thoughts for the Times on War and Death*. S.E. 14.

Freud, S. (1918). *The Taboo of Virginity*. S.E. 11.

Freud, S. (1919). *The Uncanny*. S.E. 17.

Freud, S. (1920). *Beyond the Pleasure Principle*. S.E. 18.

Freud, S. (1921). *Group Psychology and the Analysis of the Ego*. S.E. 18.

Freud, S. (1922). *Some Neurotic Mechanisms in Homosexuality, Jealousy, and Paranoia*. S.E. 18.

Freud, S. (1923). *The Ego and the Id*. S.E. 19.

Freud, S. (1924a). *Neurosis and Psychosis*. S.E. 19.

Freud, S. (1924b). *The Loss of Reality in Neurosis and Psychosis*. S.E. 19.

Freud, S. (1924c). *The Economic Problem of Masochism*. S.E. 19.

Freud, S. (1924d). *The Resistances to Psychoanalysis*. S.E. 19.

Freud, S. (1930). *Civilization and Its Discontents*. S.E. 21.

Freud, S. (1933). *Why War?* S.E. 22.

Freud, S. (1937). *Analysis Terminable and Interminable*. S.E. 23.

Freud, S. (1940). *The Splitting of the Ego in the Process of Defense*. S.E. 23.

Goldsmith, K. (2010). The Issue of Intent in the Genocide Convention and Its Effect on the Prevention and Punishment of the Crime of Genocide: Toward a Knowledge-Based Approach. *Genocide Studies and Prevention*. 5: 238–257.

Heidegger, M. (1977). *Basic Writings*. New York: Harper and Row.

Hinton, A. (ed.). (2002). *Annihilating Difference: The Anthropology of Genocide*. Berkeley: University of California Press.

Keval, N. (2016). *Racist States of Mind*. London: Routledge.

Kiernan, B. (2007). *Blood and Soil: A World History of Genocide and Extermination from Sparta to Darfur*. New Haven, CT: Yale University Press.

Klein, M. (1975). *The Psychoanalysis of Children*. New York: Delta Books.

Klein, M. (1986). *The Selected Melanie Klein*. (J. Mitchell, ed.). New York: The Free Press.

Konigsberg, R. (2014). *Hitler's Ideology: A Study in Psychoanalytic Sociology*. New York: The Library of Social Science.

Lacan, J. (1949). The Mirror Stage as Formative of the I Function. In *Ecrits*. (B. Fink, trans.). NY: Norton.

Major, R. (1999). La soif du pouvoir. In *Au commencement: La vie la mort*. Paris: Galilée.

Marcus, K. (2012). Accusation in a Mirror. *Loyola University Chicago Law Journal*. 43(2): 357–393.

Moses, A. D. (2021). *The Problems of Genocide*. Cambridge: Cambridge University Press.

Sands, P. (2016). *East West Street*. New York: Vintage.

Schabas, W. (2006). The 'Odious Scourge': Evolving Interpretations of the Crime of Genocide. *Genocide Studies and Prevention*. 1(2): 93–106.

Semelin, Jacques. 2007. *Purify and Destroy*. (Trans. C. Schoch). New York: Columbia University Press.

Southern, L., Deschner, T., and Pika, S. (2021). Lethal Coalitionary Attacks of Chimpanzees (*Pan troglodytes troglodytes*) on Gorillas (*Gorilla gorilla*) in the Wild. *Scientific Reports*. 11: 14673.

UN Convention Against Genocide. (1948). UN.org.

Waller, J. (2007). *Becoming Evil: How Ordinary People Commit Genocide and Mass Killing*. Oxford: Oxford University Press

Wyschogrod. E. (1985). *The Spirit in Ashes*. New Haven, CT: Yale University Press.

Index

For Product Safety Concerns and Information please contact our EU
representative GPSR@taylorandfrancis.com
Taylor & Francis Verlag GmbH, Kaufingerstraße 24, 80331 München, Germany

www.ingramcontent.com/pod-product-compliance
Ingram Content Group UK Ltd.
Pitfield, Milton Keynes, MK11 3LW, UK
UKHW020000200926
475702UK00015B/2394
9781032910659